Prevention

Healing Kitchen

Healthy Keto

75+ Plant-Based, Low-Carb, High-Fat Recipes

HEARST
HOME

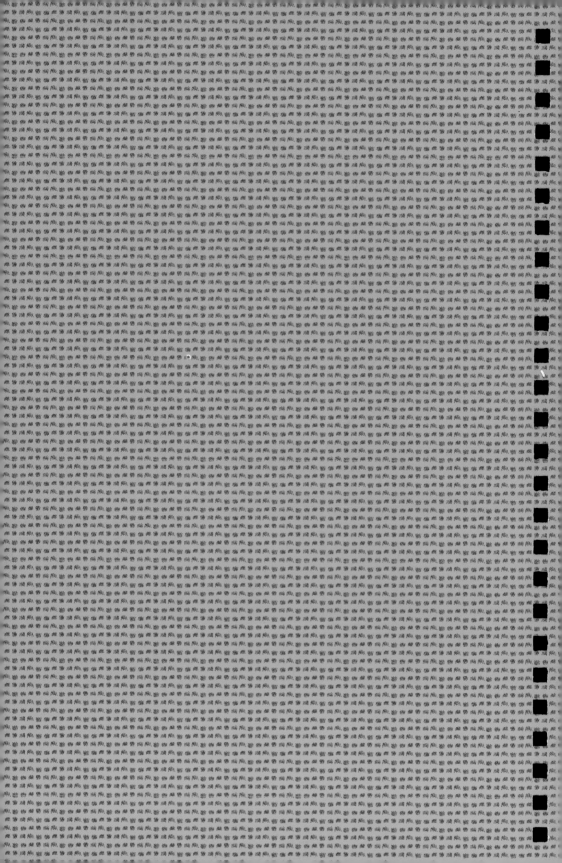

Prevention
Healing Kitchen

Contents

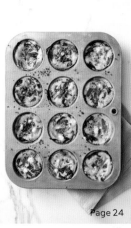

Page 24

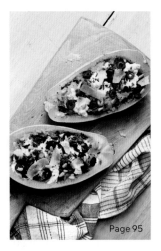

Page 95

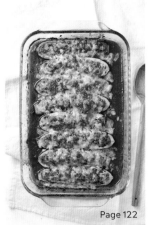

Page 122

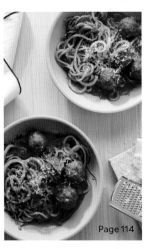

Page 114

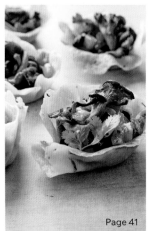

Page 41

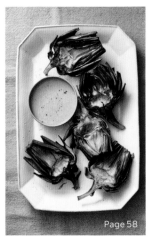

Page 58

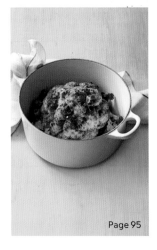

Page 95

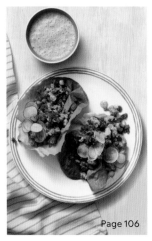

Page 106

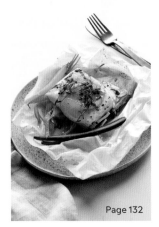

Page 132

Foreword

Though the keto diet has been used medically for nearly 100 years, it has recently attracted widespread popularity and controversy as well. Enthusiasts rave about its many potential benefits while critics balk at its over-the-top fat intake and rigid guidelines. Simultaneously, rates of obesity are on the rise—according to the World Health Organization, worldwide obesity has nearly tripled since 1975—and it's clear the business-as-usual "eat less and move more" advice is not doing enough to combat this global epidemic. Because of this, dietitians and other health professionals are increasingly challenged to find innovative ways to engage people on their wellness journey to achieve lasting results. At the same time, clinicians seek out evidence-based approaches and are wary of fad diets promising too-good-to-be-true results seemingly overnight. The keto diet, however, has been extensively studied as a unique nutrition innovation and shows encouraging results in the areas of weight loss, blood sugar control, and the prevention of cardiovascular disease and neurological disorders.

But if "keto" makes you think of downing bacon and butter exclusively, without a vegetable or fruit in sight—an approach that might appeal to some for a short period of time but becomes old very fast!—this book reveals how to healthfully implement a varied eating plan for weight loss. Difficulty sticking to the keto diet in the long term is a commonly noted challenge, so a plant-forward meal plan with a wide assortment of foods that combine fiber, antioxidants, and heart-healthy fats, among other vital nutrients, while keeping the body in a state of ketosis, is essential. The *Prevention* approach even highlights all-star ingredients that add color and interest to meals and offer myriad health benefits in addition to being keto compliant. When approached in a thoughtful way, the keto diet can be enjoyed with satisfying and delicious (and even some decadent) foods. Just look at the recipes included in this book—all dietitian approved!

—Rachel Lustgarten, MS, RD, CDN

Keto 101

The keto diet has become the most buzzed-about and controversial eating plan out there, with celebrities, dietitians, and even doctors taking positions on different sides of the fence. While Halle Berry and Al Roker are fans and have said that the diet has helped them improve their health, trainer Jillian Michaels can't get on board with this latest carb-restricting diet. So what do we think?

At *Prevention*, we believe that food is fuel, and there are many paths to weight loss. There is a responsible way to go keto, and we can help you do it. The key is to understand how the diet works and to set up your keto kitchen in a way that supports all-around health. While the 75 delicious recipes in this collection are keto compliant, they also all include one (or more!) of our 15 keto all-star ingredients (see page 16) that deliver extra benefits and nutrients for optimal health.

Please keep in mind that weight loss is a personal journey and unique to every single one of us. Though it's easy to be inspired by the success stories you hear in the news and from friends, the keto diet may not be for everyone. We encourage you to consult a doctor before starting any weight-loss regime, but if you are currently taking medications for diabetes management, it is essential that you talk to your endocrinologist before beginning the keto diet. Some medications require eating some carbs to ensure your safety.

That said, the flavorful and nourishing dishes on the following pages will fuel you not only for keto, but for life. Let's get started.

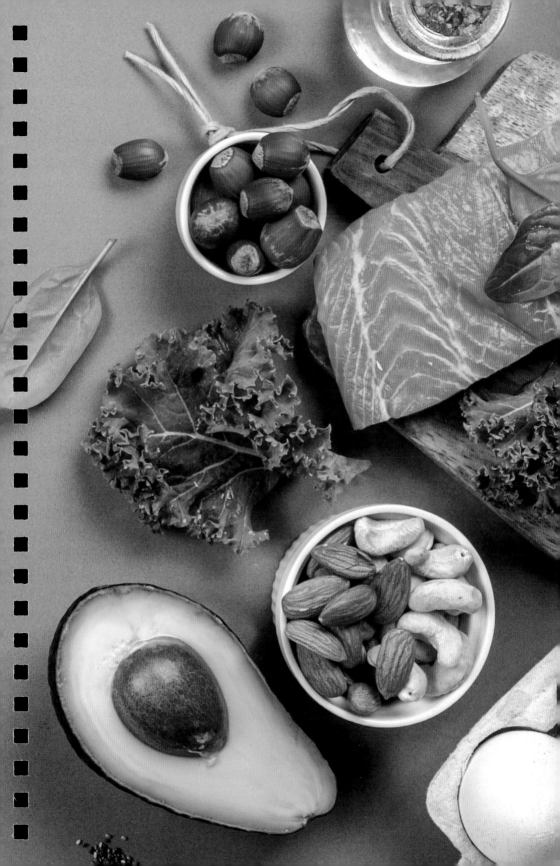

What Is the Keto Diet?

The keto diet is a high-fat, low-carb eating plan that initiates weight loss by burning fat for energy instead of the body's preferred source, glucose. As a result, your body can safely enter into ketosis, a metabolic state in which you'll break down fat—in the form of ketones—to be converted into energy. Your body's preferred source is carbs and it will always turn to those first. But when you eat fewer carbs, you begin to tap into your body's fat stores more efficiently.

The first ketogenic diets were studied in the 1920s and used to help people with epilepsy. "We have solid evidence showing that a ketogenic diet reduces seizures in children, sometimes as effectively as medication," says Marcelo Campos, MD, a primary care doctor at Harvard Vanguard. Currently, the diet has become popular in the general health world because of its ability to achieve drastic weight-loss results in a fairly quick time period.

Many keto dieters say that in addition to weight loss, they feel full longer, have more energy, and experience fewer cravings. That's largely due to the types of food you are eating: Fat contains more than twice as many calories per gram as carbs or protein (9 calories/1 gram of fat compared with 4 calories/1 gram of carb or protein), and therefore you need to eat far less to feel satiated. There's also a shift in your body's hunger and satiety hormones which may lend a hand in appetite suppression.

How Does the Diet Work?

To enter a metabolic state of ketosis, you need to be consuming about 10 percent of daily calories from dietary carbohydrates. Keto diets can vary slightly in suggested macronutrient breakdowns, but our plan recommends a moderate approach, with about 70 percent of your daily calories from healthy fats, 20 percent from protein, and 10 percent from carbs. In comparison, the recommended macro-nutrient breakdown for non-dieters is 50 percent carbs, 30 percent fat, and 20 percent protein. (See more about finding your macros on page 10.)

How Long Do I Have to Be on the Diet Before I Enter Ketosis?

Once you've started on a keto diet, your body will shift to breaking down glycogen (the storage form of carbs within your muscle and peripheral tissues) to use glucose for energy. After a few days on keto (usually about two to three days), you'll begin to tap into your body's fat stores for energy. This is the official "start" of ketosis. By eating more fat and very few calories from carbs, your metabolism will continue to use fat for fuel instead of the glucose you'd get from, say, a cracker or piece of bread.

PREVENTION'S HEALTHY KETO MACROS

70 percent* healthy fats

20 percent* proteins

10 percent* carbs

*percentages based on daily calorie intake

How Will I Know if I'm in Ketosis?

Testing for ketosis might sound complicated at first, but it's necessary in the beginning weeks of the diet to assure you are consuming the right ratio of fats, carbs, and proteins during your keto journey. There are a few methods you can take to make sure you are on target, which is important for identifying whether the diet is working correctly, or if you need to make adjustments.

An accurate method of checking for ketosis is using keto urine test strips, which give an immediate reading. Keto urine test strips are a fairly inexpensive method of testing for ketosis and can be found at pharmacies or online. When testing with the strips, it's important to be hydrated—do it after consuming liquids in the morning, for instance. If you are dehydrated, that could present a false positive.

Another test option is the blood ketone reader, which is slightly more expensive but also the most accurate. To identify that you are in proper ketosis, your blood ketone levels should be above 0.5 millimoles per liter (mmol/L) but not higher than 5.0 mmol/L.

Some people notice that they've entered ketosis by their "keto breath"—a smell or taste that could be a bit sour, fruity, and even metallic. This side effect is caused by acetone, one of the ketone bodies that is made during ketosis. It is one of the first indicators and may not be the most accurate form of evaluation. And if you are self-conscious, don't fret—it should last only the first few weeks of the keto diet and eventually will go away.

Tip Increase your fluid intake on the keto diet by at least two to four cups of water for every 30 to 60 minutes of physical activity to prevent dehydration.

What Is the Best Approach to Starting Keto?

"Although fat is the centerpiece of any keto diet, that doesn't mean you should be subsisting on butter-topped steaks," says Kristen Mancinelli, RD, author of *The Ketogenic Diet*. "A big misconception is that you should just put meat at the center of your plate and add more fat on top." To start this diet correctly and effectively, a more gradual approach is key to reduce the amount of negative keto symptoms you will experience. This will allow you to ease into the keto routine.

What do we mean by gradual? Rather than just boosting your diet with lots of unhealthy fats like butter, bacon, and cream to attain ketosis, focus on increasing healthy fats from proteins like eggs, grass-fed meat, and healthy oils.

Consuming the right amount of carbohydrates is also still important. Plant-based carbs are recommended on the gradual plan to facilitate digestion and hydration. Keto-approved veggies and fruits like some of our keto all-star ingredients (page 16) will provide fiber, which is necessary for all healthy diets and especially on keto. Having a more plant-based approach to the keto diet also helps you receive the important natural vitamins and minerals you need daily for your body to function.

As a result of eating keto, you will consume less food but still feel full because fat is not only richer in flavor than carbs but also higher in calories. Consuming more fat may also help you maintain energy thanks to nutrient density—9 kcal/g—so you'll still feel satiated sanscarbs.

How Much Should I Eat?

To follow keto successfully, it is important to track your daily macronutrients, or macros, of fat, carbs, and protein. As we've said, keto ratios can vary from plan to plan, but we recommend a calorie ratio of 70 percent fat, 20 percent protein, and 10 percent carbohydrates. Different macronutrients deliver varying degrees of energy, and your daily energy target will vary as a result of body mass and physical activity. To identify your recommended macros, you can use a keto calculator online, such as **tasteaholics .com/keto-calculator** or ketogains.com /ketogainscalculator.

When tracking macros, whether it's your first time on keto or you're a seasoned keto eater, it is essential to understand the difference between total carbs and net carbs. Net carbs account for the fiber in your food or in a recipe. For example, if a recipe contains 12 grams of carbs per serving but each serving has 4 grams of fiber, then the serving has 8 grams of net carbs. You can subtract the grams of fiber per serving because it is insoluble and therefore not absorbed by the body. It's also useful to note that fiber in your diet contributes to feeling fuller longer and also aids in easier digestion (a common concern of keto eaters).

What Are Some of the Challenges?

As with any eating plan, there's always an adjustment phase with the keto diet, and some negative symptoms can arise. "Keto breath" (page 9) is one example.

Another symptom you might experience is an urgency to use the restroom. Carbohydrates retain fluid and electrolytes in the body (imagine a piece of bread absorbing water versus an egg). When you decrease the amount of carbohydrates in your diet, extra water is removed by way of urine. This makes it extremely important to consume plenty of water and electrolytes during the keto diet to avoid dehydration, kidney stones, fatigue, and constipation.

Hydration is also particularly important when starting the diet to avoid the "keto flu." Not related to influenza, keto flu involves symptoms (see below) that can arise one to two days after beginning the diet. To try to avoid these symptoms, hydration and consumption of electrolytes, including important minerals such as sodium, potassium, and calcium, are important, as is taking a dietary supplement to help replenish vitamins and minerals lost from consuming fewer starchy vegetables, fruits, and grains.

Certain fats consumed in the keto diet can have increased levels of saturated fats, which raise "bad" LDL cholesterol

KETO FLU SYMPTOMS

Bad breath	Weakness or fatigue	Headache	Nausea
Muscle cramps	Diarrhea or constipation	Skin rashes	Mood swings

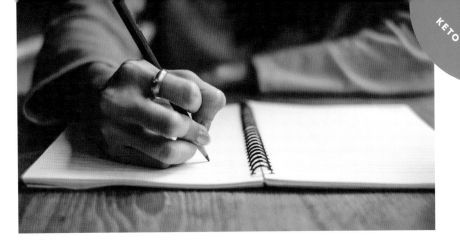

SET UP FOR SUCCESS: FOOD/MOOD JOURNAL

Maintaining ketosis is an important part of doing keto. Falling out of ketosis can cause a hormonal shift in the body that can make you even hungrier than you were before starting the diet and reverse your weight-loss goal. Keeping a mood and food journal to track symptoms as well as the macronutrients you're eating can help you sustain your keto journey. While you may believe you're eating right, memory is selective. Plus, it's easy to overlook bites, licks, and tastes, but they quickly add up! The solution? Write them down. In a landmark Kaiser Permanente study of more than 2,000 dieters, keeping a food diary turned out to be the best predictor of whether people would lose weight. Similarly, when tracking your daily meals, keeping a food and mood journal will help you understand your eating patterns in order to maintain ketosis. Tracking how you feel before and after a meal, in coordination with daily macros, helps you identify "keto flu" or "keto breath" and handle these diet challenges with increased hydration and vitamin/mineral supplements.

and cause atherosclerosis, the buildup of fats and cholesterol in the arteries. Fat can also be more difficult to digest and absorb than carbs and protein. For those with type 2 diabetes or who rely on exogenous insulin or oral hypoglycemics, it's important to understand the health effects of reducing the amount of carbs and increasing the fat in your diet for proper management of your condition.

As with all diets, it's important to consult a doctor when considering the switch to the keto diet, especially if you're at risk for high cholesterol, high blood pressure, type 2 diabetes, heart disease, lifestyle-related cancers, Alzheimer's disease, or any GI disorders, such as pancreatitis, cholecystitis, irritable bowel syndrome, or inflammatory bowel disease. And a restrictive plan like keto is a definite no-no if you have a history of disordered eating, if you're pregnant or lactating, or if you're taking exogenous insulin or oral hypoglycemic agents for the management of type 1 or type 2 diabetes.

Set Up for Success

When prepping for a new meal or diet plan, one of the first keys to success is planning your kitchen and pantry to keep you on track.

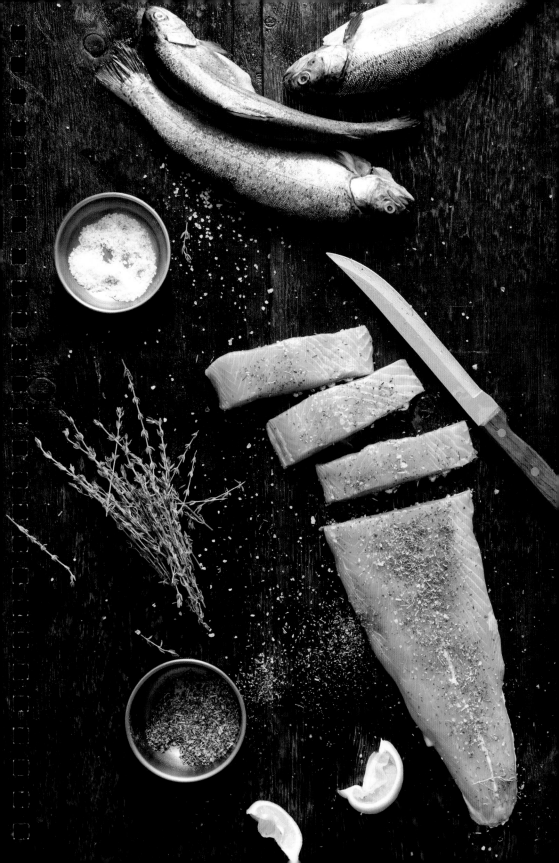

Shop for Keto-Friendly Foods

When shopping, be sure to read the labels! Look at the nutritional information on packages to see carb content, sugar, and additives such as sugar alcohols (they can be easily spotted as ingredients ending in "-ol"). Delicious ingredients to stock up on in your kitchen include:

Fats: olive oil, coconut oil, butter, ghee, avocado oil, MCT oil, avocados
Proteins: beef, poultry, pork, lamb, turkey, eggs, fish
Non-starchy veggies: leafy greens, bell peppers, cruciferous veggies (broccoli, cabbage, cauliflower, Brussels sprouts), cucumbers, eggplant, garlic, mushrooms, olives, onions, tomatoes, zucchini
Sweeteners: stevia, erythritol, sugar-free maple syrup
Beverages: water, coffee, tea
Broths: chicken, beef, bone
Herbs and spices: any fresh or dried herbs and spices
Pickled and fermented foods: pickles, kimchi, sauerkraut
Low-carb condiments: mayo, mustard, pesto, sriracha

Keep the Rule of Moderation

Some foods are okay on the keto diet as long as you are tracking your carbs. These include:

Full-fat dairy: milk, cheese, yogurt
Medium-starchy veggies: carrots, beets, parsnips, peas, artichokes
Legumes: such as peanuts
Nuts and seeds: almonds, cashews, walnuts, pumpkin seeds, sunflower seeds
Fruits: berries, melons, other low-sugar fruits

Tip When thinking about keto-friendly beverages, stick to drinks that have no sugar, such as water, coffee, or tea. When it comes to alcohol, avoid beer, low-carb beer, and wine because of the carb count of 3 grams per serving. Try pure spirits like vodka, gin, and tequila—they have zero carbs!

Be Aware of These Foods

Remove high-carb foods from your refrigerator and pantry and you are already on your way to earning a keto gold medal. These aren't all necessarily foods that are bad for you, just ones that won't help you on a keto-specific journey. Some examples of items to discard:

All types of sugar: honey, agave, maple syrup, and beverages like soda, fruit juice, and energy drinks
Grains: wheat, oats, all types of rice, corn
Legumes: lentils, peas, beans, chickpeas
All foods made with flour: breads, cracker, pastas
Processed foods and oils: anything that comes in a bag or a box, salad dressings, dips
Hight-carb fruits: bananas, grapes, mangoes, dates, dried cranberries, dried cherries

Tools for the Task

Keeping recipes simple and easy to prepare will help you resist outside food temptations. You will need the usual cooking tools like pots, pans, and skillets. Other equipment to help you prepare these recipes includes:

1. **Sharp knives:** They're key for any good cook. A chef's knife, a paring knife, and a serrated knife will help you master the chopping and prep like a pro.
2. **Food scale & measuring spoons:** Precision is important to maintaining the diet and measuring your macronutrient ingredients correctly.
3. **Food processor:** Helps with pureeing dips and sauces and chopping cauliflower rice.
4. **Blender:** For easy morning smoothies, shakes, and even soups!
5. **Spiralizer:** Turn any low-carb veggie into an easy carb substitute by making it instantly into noodles.

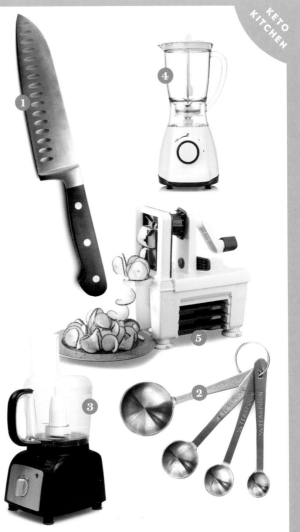

Meal Planning Is Essential

Now that you have your refrigerator and pantry stocked, your meal planning just got that much easier. If you have the ingredients at hand and know what you're making, you will be on track. To start the keto plan for weight loss, you must break down your macronutrient intake properly. You can use an online keto calculator (page 10). When planning recipes for your own keto meal program, if the macros are not matching up with your daily needs, look at the serving size of a recipe and go from there—you may need half a serving or double a serving to meet your daily macro needs. After a few days, test whether you have begun ketosis with the keto urine test strips (page 9), and you will be able to regulate your nutrient levels from there. Once you get the hang of it, you will find your own personal keto routine, and meals will become easier and easier.

15 Keto All-Stars

The grocery store can become very overwhelming when you're trying a diet or planning meals in a new way. This is our list of keto all-star ingredients that have incredible health benefits beyond the keto diet. Packed with essential vitamins, minerals, and other important nutrients such as fiber, healthy fats, and antioxidants, these foods are beneficial to your overall health, and others in your household will reap their benefits if you are making keto compliant meals for all.

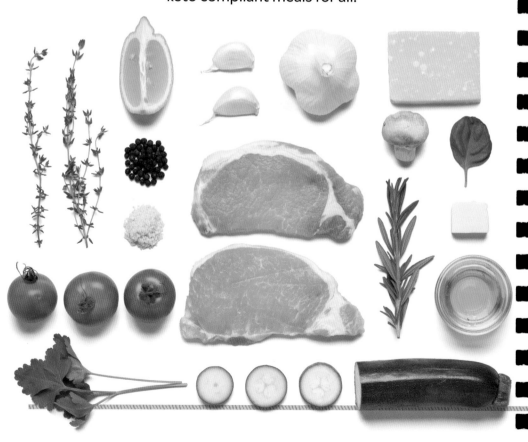

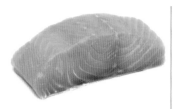
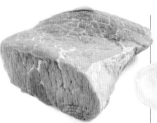
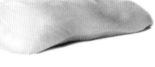

SALMON AND OTHER SEAFOOD

Salmon is a rich source of vitamin D and one of the best sources of omega-3s you can find. Other seafood such as tuna, shrimp, and sardines also contain these essential fatty acids that have a wide range of impressive health benefits—from preventing heart disease, to smoothing your skin, to aiding weight loss and bloating, to boosting your mood. Omega-3s also slow the rate of digestion, making you feel fuller longer, which means salmon and other seafood are a perfect source of fat and lean protein on the keto diet.

LEAN BEEF

Lean beef is one of the best-absorbed sources of iron available. Adding as little as one ounce of beef per day can make a big difference in the body's ability to absorb iron from other sources, says Mary J. Kretsch, PhD, a researcher at the USDA-ARS Western Human Nutrition Research Center in Davis, California. Beef also packs plenty of zinc and B vitamins, which help your body convert food into energy. If you can afford to splurge, choose grass-fed beef. Compared with grain-fed beef, it has twice the concentration of vitamin E, a powerful brain-boosting antioxidant. It's also high in omega-3 fatty acids.

CHICKEN BREAST

It may not be a trendy superfood, but chicken breast is a rich source of protein. Chicken breasts are also a great source of phosphorous—important for strong bones and teeth—as well as vitamin B3 (a.k.a. niacin), which helps control high blood pressure and prevents hardening of the arteries. One serving also contains 25 percent of the vitamin B6 you need each day to maintain proper brain and immune system function. This lean protein is essential to any diet.

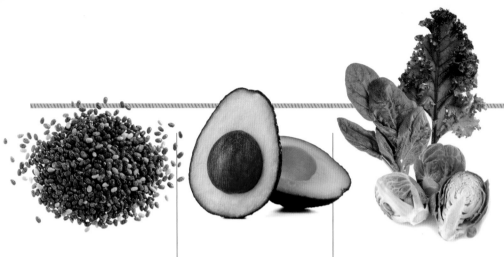

CHIA SEEDS

Chia seeds are a great source of protein, omega-3s, and fiber. They also contain good amounts of healthy antioxidants, as well as calcium, zinc, magnesium, and iron—all important for your health. Toss a small handful into the Green Light Smoothie (page 32), use them to replace poppy seeds in Poppy Seed-Cheddar Bark (page 51), add them as a healthful topping on salads, or make them the star of your breakfast in Classic Creamy Chia Pudding (page 26).

AVOCADO

These smooth, buttery fruits are a wonderful source of not only monounsaturated fats (MUFAs) but other important nutrients as well. Avocados contain heart-smart nutrients, such as soluble fiber, vitamin E, folate, and potassium. Though fat is key on keto, avocados are still calorie-dense, so be sure to watch your portion sizes.

LEAFY GREENS

Dark leafy greens, such as kale, spinach, and Swiss chard, tend to top health experts' best foods lists. Bursting with vitamins A, K, and C, kale is a great source of calcium, iron, magnesium, and potassium. Spinach has serious health muscles: It's a rich source of lutein, which may prevent heart attacks. Spinach is also rich in iron, folate, and B vitamins that prevent birth defects. And Brussels sprouts are a cruciferous vegetable that features sulfur compounds called glucosinolates that are shown to help lower the risk for several types of cancer and detoxify our bodies.

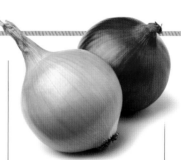
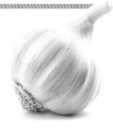

GARLIC

Garlic is a flavor essential and a health superstar in its own right. The onion's relative contains more than 70 active phytochemicals, including allicin, which studies have shown may decrease high blood pressure. Allicin also fights infection and bacteria. Plus, garlic adds a whole lot of flavor with very few calories. The key to healthier garlic: Crush the cloves, and let them stand for up to 30 minutes before cooking; that activates and preserves their heart-protecting compounds.

ONIONS

They're champs when it comes to polyphenols and flavonoids, both of which are linked to lower oxidative stress and reduced cancer risk. An onion's sulfur compounds can also help control diabetes symptoms and protect your heart from disease. And similar to garlic, onions can add a nice bite when used raw or a great aroma when cooked.

Tip **The outermost layers tend to hold more healthy nutrients.**

TOMATOES

Tomatoes are our most common source of lycopene, an antioxidant that may protect against heart disease and breast cancer. Lucky for keto eaters, this fruit has four grams of carbs and two grams of sugar per half-cup serving, making them an all-star ingredient to enjoy frequently. For a healthier side dish, quarter plum tomatoes and coat with olive oil, garlic powder, salt, and pepper. Roast in a 400°F oven for 20 minutes and serve with roast chicken.

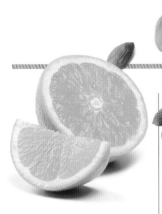

CITRUS

Loaded with vitamin C, oranges are also solid sources of folate—important for cell maintenance and repair. They contain potassium and vitamins B1 and A, which are essential for vision and immune function. And the pectin in oranges absorbs unhealthy cholesterol from the other foods you eat. Along with its impressive concentrations of vitamin C, lemon contains flavonoid compounds shown to have anti-cancer properties. But lemons may be healthiest in a supporting role: Add a little to your tea and your body will absorb more of the drink's healthy antioxidants, finds research from Purdue University. Plus, the citric acid and vitamin C in limes can help alleviate inflammation or arthritis, maintain clear skin, and improve heart health.

NUTS AND NUT BUTTERS

USDA researchers say that eating 1.5 ounces of tree nuts daily can reduce your risk of heart disease and diabetes. Walnuts are rich in omega-3s, while hazelnuts contain arginine, an amino acid that may lower blood pressure. An ounce of almonds has as many heart-healthy polyphenols as a cup of green tea. The key is moderation, since nuts are high in calories and some varieties are higher in carbs than others (see page 44). Enjoying nut butter is also encouraged, since they provide magnesium, calcium, and B vitamins that help muscle and nuerological function. Make sure to choose the unsweetened variety with no added sugar.

EGGS

Egg yolks provide many essential but hard-to-get nutrients, including choline, which is linked to lower rates of breast cancer. One yolk supplies 25 percent of your daily need and also provides antioxidants that may help decrease your risk of macular degeneration and cataracts. In fact, research shows that eating one whole egg a day won't raise your risk of heart attack or stroke. Plus, since they are high in fat (5 grams of fat in one egg), they make a great start to your day when on the keto diet.

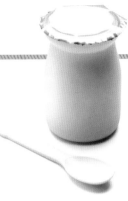

GREEK YOGURT

Yogurt is a premium source of calcium, and it's also rich in immune-boosting probiotics (see more on page 47). But the next time you hit the yogurt aisle, pick up the Greek kind. Compared with regular yogurt, it has twice the protein. When on the keto diet, look for full-fat, plain, unsweetened varieties.

MUSHROOMS

Compounds found in mushrooms have been linked to lowered cholesterol levels, and their antioxidant content may help decrease your risk of some cancers, according to the American Cancer Society. Mushrooms also contain selenium and are a plant-based form of vitamin D, which will help boost immunity overall. Plus, they are naturally low-carb!

OLIVE OIL

Olive oil is packed with heart-healthy MUFAs, which help lower "bad" LDL cholesterol and raise "good" HDL cholesterol. It's rich in antioxidants that can help reduce the risk of cancer and other chronic diseases, like Alzheimer's. Look for extra-virgin oils for the most antioxidants and flavor. This oil will become your go-to on the keto diet, but for a list of other keto-friendly oils, see page 99.

Tip **Each recipe featured in the upcoming chapters has at least one of these all-star keto ingredients! To identify them easily, we have added a star next to them in the ingredient list. ✪**

Chapter 1

Breakfast

A good or bad breakfast is often an indicator of how you will eat for the rest of the day. To attain and maintain proper ketosis, it is important to always keep breakfast on track. A healthy keto breakfast begins with a high amount of healthy fats as well as a reasonable amount of protein to keep you full all morning. Add in some fiber for good digestion and keto is easy.

Breakfast should never be difficult! Try the Green Light Smoothie or the Cheddar, Pepper & Avocado Eggs for a quick on-the-go solution. Make the Spinach & Pepper Mini Frittatas or the Classic Creamy Chia Pudding the night before for a breakfast that is ready to eat in the morning. On weekends, try the Avocado, Ham & Egg Cups or the Tomato & Egg Stacks for a meal the whole family will love.

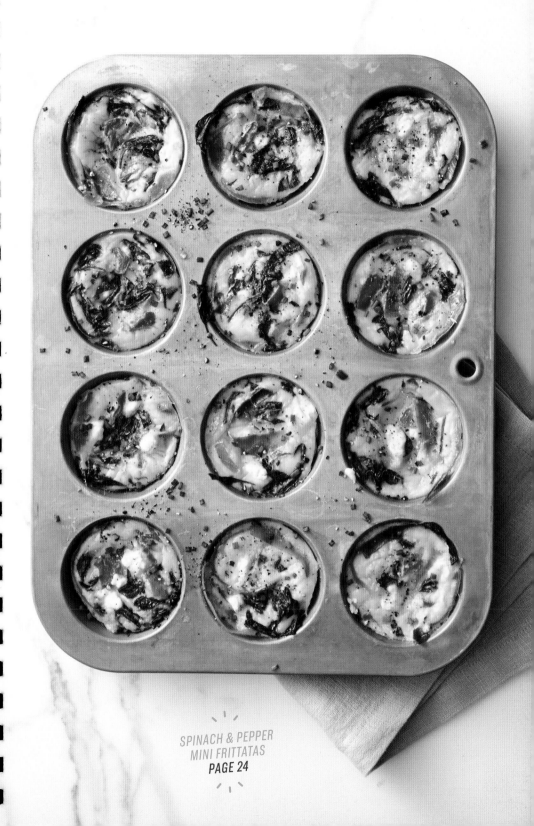

SPINACH & PEPPER
MINI FRITTATAS
PAGE 24

Spinach & Pepper Mini Frittatas

Active time: 25 minutes
Total time: 45 minutes
Makes: 12 servings

→ With 1 gram of carbs, 5 grams of fat, and 6 grams of protein, eggs are an essential keto breakfast food. The protein keeps you full all morning and the "good" type of cholesterol, known as HDL, helps to reduce the risk of heart attack and stroke. Plus, the added fiber from the baby spinach results in only 1 net carb.

INGREDIENTS
- 1 tablespoon olive oil
  1 large red bell pepper, cut into ¼-inch pieces
  Kosher salt and pepper
- 2 scallions, chopped
- 6 large eggs
  ½ cup milk
- 1 5-ounce package baby spinach, chopped
  ¼ cup fresh goat cheese, crumbled

1. Heat oven to 350°F. Spray a 12-cup muffin pan with nonstick cooking spray.

2. Heat olive oil in a large skillet on medium. Add red bell pepper and ⅛ teaspoon each salt and pepper. Cover and cook, stirring occasionally, until tender, 6 to 8 minutes. Remove from heat and stir in scallions.

3. In a large bowl, beat together eggs, milk, ¼ teaspoon salt, and ⅛ teaspoon pepper. Stir in spinach and red pepper mixture.

4. Divide batter among muffin pan cups (about ¼ cup for each muffin), top with goat cheese, and bake until just set in the center, 20 to 25 minutes. (Even when set, tops of frittatas may look wet from the spinach.)

5. Let cool on a wire rack 5 minutes, then remove frittatas from pan. Serve warm.

PER SERVING: 65 calories, 4.5 g fat (1.5 g saturated fat), 4 g protein, 120 mg sodium, 2 g carbohydrates, 1 g sugars (0 g added sugars), 1 g fiber

Summer Squash Frittata

Active time: 10 minutes
Total time: 35 minutes
Makes: 4 servings

→ A combination of zucchini and yellow squash creates a visual feast. Summer squashes are rich in antioxidants and carotenoids like beta-carotene, which benefits your eyes, skin, and heart. Don't peel your summer squash either; the skin contains the most antioxidants. Use a mandoline to thinly slice the summer squash for this recipe.

INGREDIENTS

1½ pounds summer squash, very thinly sliced
Kosher salt
✪ 8 large eggs
4 ounces Gruyère cheese, shredded
¾ cup whole milk
✪ 2 green onions, thinly sliced
¼ teaspoon ground black pepper

1. Heat oven to 375°F. In a bowl, toss squash with ½ teaspoon salt; let stand 10 minutes, then gently squeeze very dry.

2. In a bowl, whisk together eggs, cheese, milk, green onions, pepper, and ¼ teaspoon salt.

3. Heat a 10-inch oven-safe nonstick skillet on medium. Add the egg mixture. Stir in squash. Cook, occasionally stirring and pulling back the edges, 2 minutes, or until the bottom begins to set. Cook, without stirring, 3 more minutes.

4. Transfer the skillet to the preheated oven; bake 20 to 25 minutes, or until set.

PER SERVING: 320 calories, 21 g fat (10 g saturated), 25 g protein, 690 mg sodium, 9 g carbohydrates, 9 g sugars (0 g added sugars), 2 g fiber

 Tip You can swap in an equal amount of another cheese for the Gruyère if you like.

Classic Creamy Chia Pudding

Active time: 10 minutes
Total time: 10 minutes plus chilling
Makes: 4 servings

→ Chia seeds are an excellent, nutritious addition to your keto diet, and because they expand in water, they can also help you stay hydrated throughout the day. Chia seeds are gluten-free and contain alpha-linolenic acid (ALA), which is a plant-based omega-3 fatty acid that helps fight inflammation. Plus, they contain a decent amount of protein for such a small amount of seeds, perfect for maintaining ketosis.

INGREDIENTS
- ✪ 5 tablespoons chia seeds
- 1–2 drops liquid stevia
- 1⅓ cups milk or unsweetened plant-based milk

To a small bowl, add chia seeds, liquid stevia, and milk or unsweetened plant-based milk. Whisk to combine and cover. Refrigerate overnight. Can keep in the fridge for up to 4 days.

PER SERVING: 113 calories, 7 g fat (2 g saturated fat), 5 g protein, 37 g sodium, 9 g carbohydrates, 4 g sugar (0 g added sugar), 5 g fiber

VARIATIONS

BLUEBERRY-COCONUT
Make Classic Chia Pudding, replacing milk with 3 cups coconut milk. To serve, stir in ¼ teaspoon lemon zest per serving and top each with 1 tablespoon blueberries.

PB&J
Make Classic Chia Pudding. To serve, stir in 1 tablespoon peanut butter per serving and top each with a sliced strawberry.

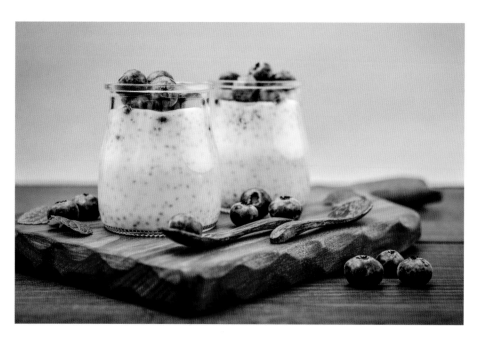

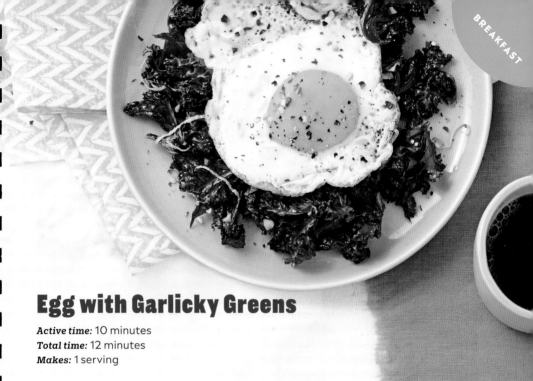

Egg with Garlicky Greens

Active time: 10 minutes
Total time: 12 minutes
Makes: 1 serving

→ Using dark leafy greens, such as kale, spinach, and Swiss chard, provides a boost of fiber to your diet and helps you avoid constipation during keto. Better yet, greens like these deliver a source of calcium and iron as well as vitamins A, C, and K to promote healthy bones and fight infection. For an easy shortcut in the morning, use the baby varieties of dark leafy greens, such as baby kale or baby spinach, and forget the chopping!

INGREDIENTS
- 2 teaspoons olive oil
- ½ teaspoon minced garlic
- 1 ½ cups chopped dark leafy greens
- Salt and pepper
- 1 egg
- Red pepper flakes, for topping
- Lemon zest, for topping

1. Heat 1 teaspoon olive oil in a small nonstick skillet. Sauté garlic and greens until wilted, about 3 minutes; season with salt and pepper and remove from pan.

2. In same skillet, add 1 teaspoon olive oil and fry egg on medium-high for 4 minutes.

3. Top greens with fried egg; garnish with red pepper flakes and lemon zest before serving.

PER SERVING: 166 calories, 14 g fat (3 g saturated fat), 7 g protein, 320 mg sodium, 3 g carbohydrates, 1 g sugars (0 g added sugars), 1 g fiber

Tip Many grocery stores sell pre-chopped dark leafy greens in the produce section alongside lettuces. Be sure to choose dark leafy greens to receive their strong nutrient contents!

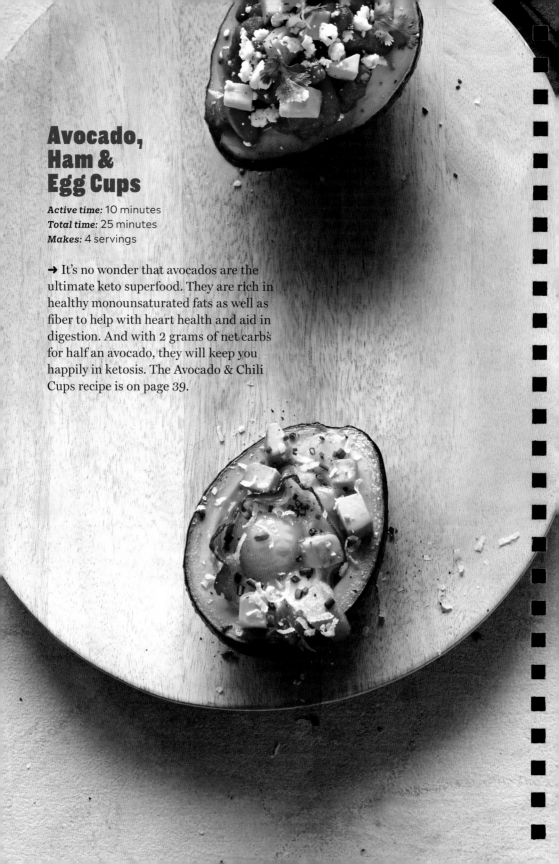

Avocado, Ham & Egg Cups

Active time: 10 minutes
Total time: 25 minutes
Makes: 4 servings

➜ It's no wonder that avocados are the ultimate keto superfood. They are rich in healthy monounsaturated fats as well as fiber to help with heart health and aid in digestion. And with 2 grams of net carbs for half an avocado, they will keep you happily in ketosis. The Avocado & Chili Cups recipe is on page 39.

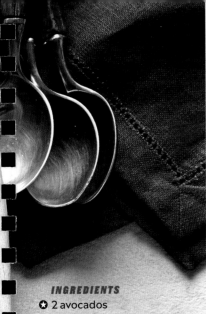

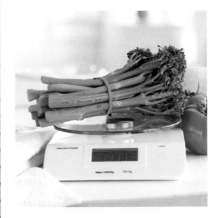

INGREDIENTS

- ❂ 2 avocados
- 2 slices ham
- ❂ 4 eggs
- Salt and pepper
- Chopped chives, for topping
- Parmesan, for topping

1. Heat oven to 425°F. Halve avocados and scoop out ⅓ of the flesh from each half around the pit's indentation. Dice scooped flesh and set aside.

2. Halve ham slices and fit a slice into each avocado half to form a cup. Place avocado halves on a rimmed baking sheet. Carefully pour 1 egg into each cup. Season to taste with salt and pepper and bake until egg is set but yolk is still runny, about 15 minutes. Remove from oven and top with chives, Parmesan, and diced avocado.

PER SERVING: 267 calories, 21.5 g fat (4.5 g saturated fat), 12 g protein, 513 mg sodium, 9 g carbohydrates, 1 g sugars (0 g added sugars), 7 g fiber

WHY FIBER IS GOOD FOR YOU

When counting your macros, it's more important to track your net carbs than total carbs because the net figure accounts for a very important nutrient: fiber. Essential for a healthy and balanced diet, fiber is a super nutrient with many powerful benefits, such as slowing the rate at which sugar is absorbed into the bloodstream and aiding in digestion. It also helps keep you feeling full longer, which assists in weight control and loss. Fiber recommendations vary by age and gender and also decrease with age. General guidelines suggest 14 grams of fiber per 1,000 calories in your diet. Below, personal fiber needs for women and men in different age categories are provided:

WOMEN

19 to 30 years old = 28 grams per day
31 to 50 years old = 25 grams per day
51 and older = 22 grams per day

MEN

19 to 30 years old = 34 grams per day
31 to 50 years old = 31 grams per day
51 and older = 28 grams per day

When eating keto, it can be hard to maintain healthy fiber levels as many hearty whole grains and beans provide a great source of fiber but are not allowed on the diet. That said, keto-friendly foods such as nuts, seeds, vegetables, and fruits also contain important sources of fiber.

Cheddar, Pepper & Avocado Eggs

Active time: 8 minutes
Total time: 10 minutes
Makes: 1 serving

→ Yes, finally a diet that encourages eating cheese in moderation. Cheese is high in fat, low in carbs, and also contains protein, making it just what you need on the keto diet. Plus, one ounce of Cheddar cheese contains 20 percent of your Reference Daily Intake of calcium, which is great for bone health and may even reduce the risk of cancer, diabetes, and high blood pressure.

INGREDIENTS
1 ounce extra-sharp Cheddar, coarsely grated
✪ 1 scallion, finely chopped
1 ounce ham, cut into ½-inch pieces
✪ 2 large eggs
1 tablespoon milk
Salt and pepper
⅛ chopped red bell pepper, for topping
✪ ⅛ avocado, for topping

1. Place half the Cheddar, half the scallions, and half the ham in a 10- to 12-ounce jar. Add eggs, milk, and a pinch each salt and pepper.

2. Screw lid on tightly and shake the jar until the ingredients are well mixed, about 20 seconds. Remove lid and microwave for 60 seconds, then in 15-second intervals until just set.

3. Remove from the microwave and top eggs with chopped red bell pepper, avocado, and remaining Cheddar, scallions, and ham.

PER SERVING: 356 calories, 25 g fat (10.5 g saturated fat), 26 g protein, 788 mg sodium, 6 g carbohydrates, 2 g sugars (0 g added sugars), 2 g fiber

Boursin, Bacon & Spinach Eggs

Active time: 5 minutes
Total time: 9 minutes
Makes: 1 serving

→ You may have heard that the keto diet means you can eat a lot of bacon. At *Prevention*, we believe that while bacon is definitely high in fat, which helps to maintain ketosis, it should be eaten—and enjoyed—in moderation. Bacon is a processed meat that undergoes curing and as a result has been linked to causing high blood pressure and diseases such as cancer and diabetes.

INGREDIENTS
2 slices bacon
✪ ½ cup baby spinach
1 ounce Boursin cheese, crumbled
2 chives, finely chopped
✪ 2 large eggs
1 tablespoon milk
Salt and pepper

1. Place bacon between 2 sheets of paper towel on a plate. Microwave until crispy, 2 to 3 minutes. Let cool, then break into small pieces.

2. Place baby spinach, half the Boursin, and chives in a 10- to 12-ounce jar. Add eggs, milk, and a pinch each salt and pepper.

3. Screw lid on tightly and shake the jar until the ingredients are well mixed, about 20 seconds. Remove lid and microwave for 60 seconds, then in 15-second intervals until just set.

4. Remove from the microwave and top eggs with remaining Boursin and chives.

PER SERVING: 364 calories, 28 g fat (13.5 g saturated fat), 22 g protein, 746 mg sodium, 4 g carbohydrates, 2 g sugars (0 g added sugars), 1 g fiber

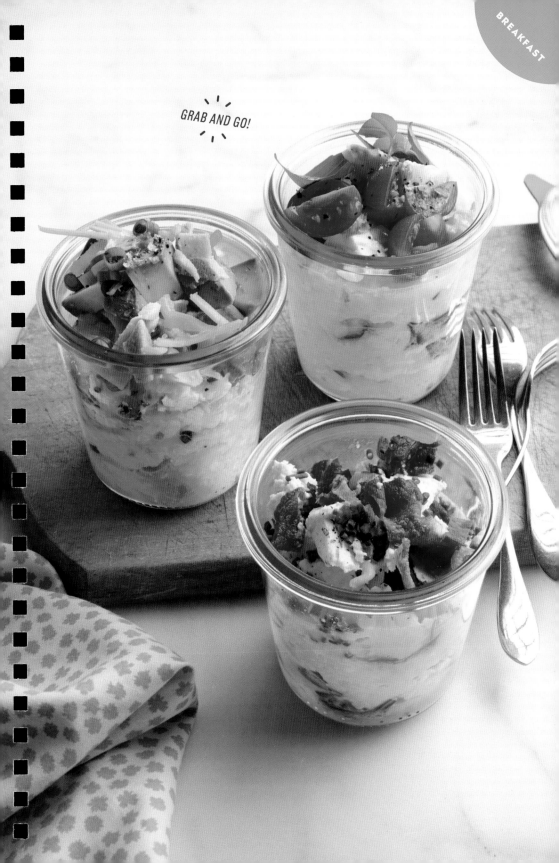

GRAB AND GO!

Tomato, Mozzarella & Basil Eggs

Active time: 5 minutes
Total time: 7 minutes
Makes: 1 serving

→ Here's a take on Caprese salad for breakfast! Fresh mozzarella offers beneficial minerals such as calcium and phosphorous. See photo page 31.

INGREDIENTS

1 ounce fresh mozzarella, chopped into small pieces
3 large basil leaves, roughly chopped
✪ 2 large eggs
1 tablespoon milk
Salt and pepper
✪ 3 cherry or grape tomatoes

1. Place half the mozzarella and half the basil in a 10- to 12-ounce jar. Add eggs, milk, and a pinch each salt and pepper.

2. Screw lid on tightly and shake the jar until the ingredients are well mixed, about 20 seconds. Remove lid and microwave for 60 seconds, then in 15-second intervals until just set.

3. Remove from the microwave and top eggs with tomatoes and remaining mozzarella and basil.

PER SERVING: 242 calories, 17 g fat (7.5 g saturated fat), 19 g protein, 281 mg sodium, 4 g carbohydrates, 2 g sugars (0 g added sugars), 1 g fiber

---

Green Light Smoothie

Total: 10 minutes
Makes: 1 serving

→ This is our kind of "juice": a savory powerhouse that uses spinach and avocado to create a green-machine smoothie. The spinach is rich in iron and folate, for blood cells and avocado provides the healthy fat and a silky texture.

INGREDIENTS

¾ cup unsweetened canned coconut milk
✪ ½ small (6 ounce) avocado
✪ 1 cup baby spinach
✪ 1 tablespoon fresh lime juice
1 tablespoon protein powder
¾ cup ice (6 cubes)
½ teaspoon matcha green tea powder (optional)

1. Put coconut milk, avocado, spinach, lime juice, protein powder, ice, and matcha powder in a blender and blend until smooth.

2. Pour into a glass and serve immediately.

PER SERVING: 505 calories, 46 g fat (34 g saturated fat), 18 g protein, 93 mg sodium, 14 g carbohydrates, 1 g sugars (0 g added sugars), 6 g fiber

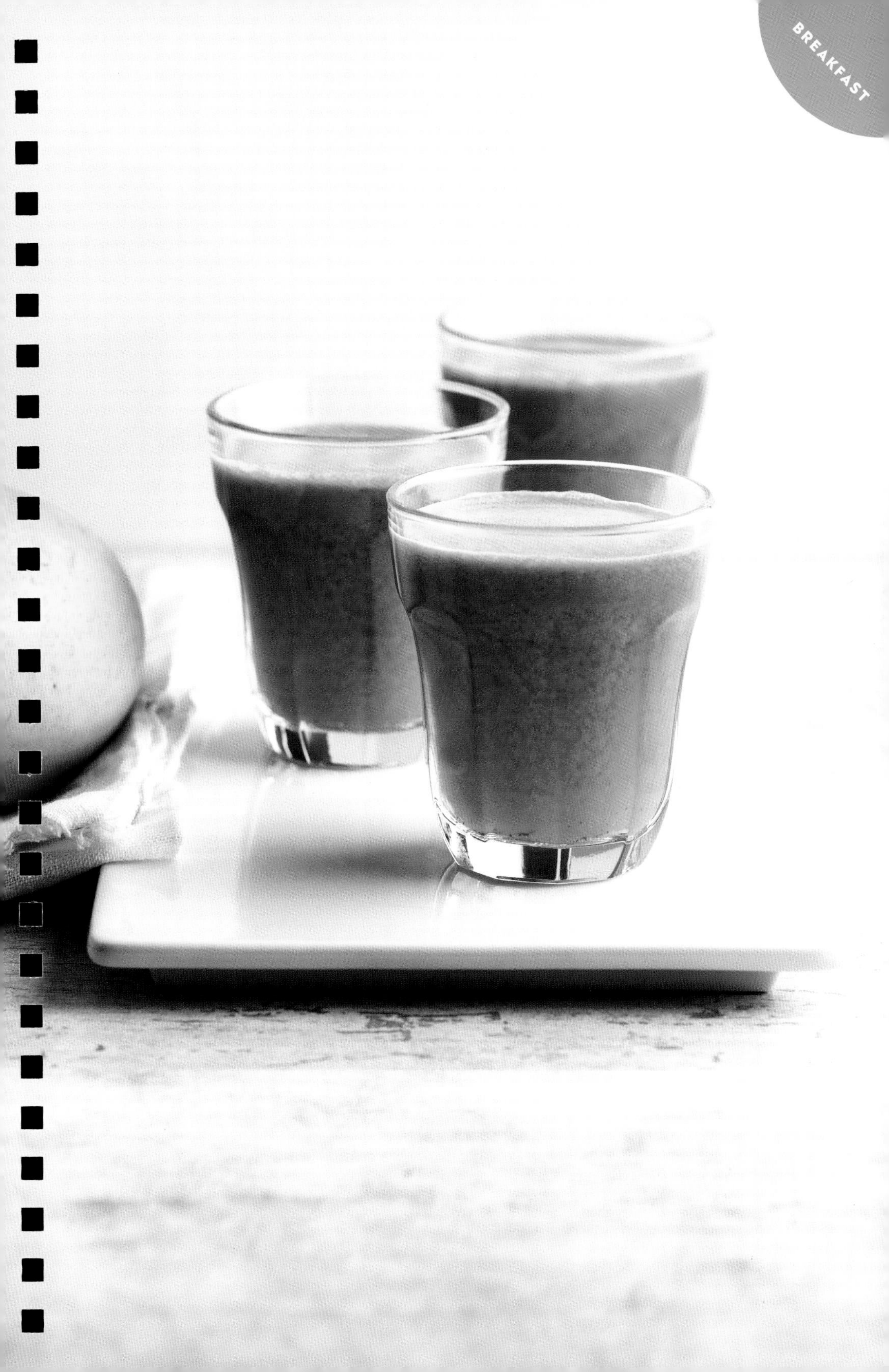

Tomato & Egg Stacks

Active time: 10 minutes
Total time: 50 minutes
Makes: 4 servings

➜ Nothing tastes better than a fresh, juicy tomato—especially in the summer. And when baked, its naturally sweet flavor is enhanced. Tomatoes contain lycopene, an antioxidant that can help protect against breast cancer. Tomatoes are also a good source of vitamin C and potassium, keeping you regular.

INGREDIENTS

- ✪ 3 teaspoons olive oil
- 2 teaspoons chopped thyme leaves
- ✪ 1 large yellow onion, thinly sliced
- ½ teaspoon kosher salt
- ✪ 1 large beefsteak tomato, sliced into 4 rounds
- 3 ounces coarsely grated smoked mozzarella
- 4 slices reduced-sodium ham (about 4 ounces), sliced into strips
- ✪ 4 large eggs

1. Heat oven to 400°F. Heat 2 teaspoons olive oil in a medium nonstick skillet on medium-high. Add thyme, onion, and salt. Cook, stirring, until onion is soft, about 6 minutes. Reduce heat to low and continue to cook, stirring occasionally, until onion is golden brown, about 20 minutes. Transfer onion to a bowl.

2. Lightly coat a rimmed baking sheet with cooking spray. Arrange tomato slices in an even layer and top with cheese and onion. Bake until cheese is melted, 5 to 7 minutes. Meanwhile, in same skillet heat 1 teaspoon olive oil on medium-high. Add ham and cook until crisp, about 2 minutes. Poach or fry eggs. Top each tomato slice with ham and an egg before serving. Season with additional thyme, if desired.

PER SERVING: 231 calories, 15 g fat (5.5 g saturated fat), 18 g protein, 773 mg sodium, 5 g carbohydrates, 3 g sugars (0 g added sugars), 1 g fiber

Tip In July and August or peak tomato season, try experimenting with different varieties of ripe tomatoes at the market, like heirlooms. These rainbow tomatoes are very sweet and juicy in comparison with regular tomatoes, and still boast the health benefits.

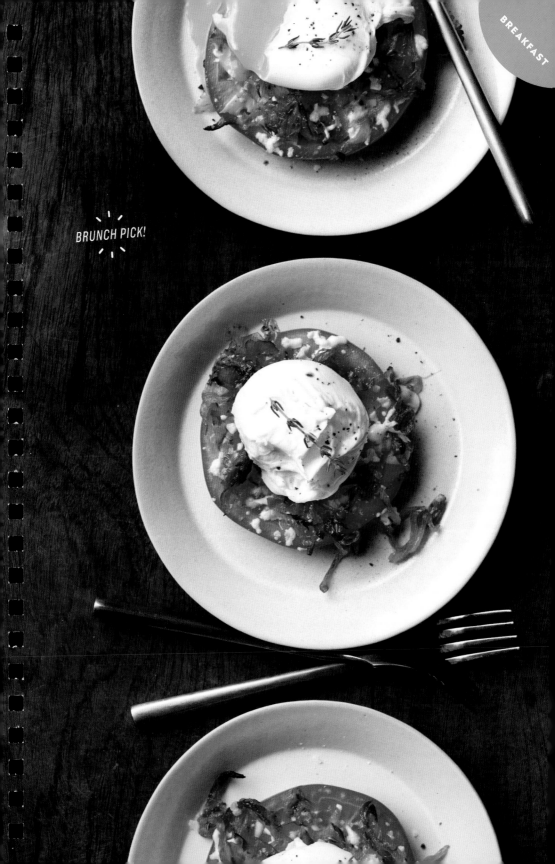

BRUNCH PICK!

Chapter 2

Apps & Snacks

Let's face it: Snacking is hard to completely eliminate. But it's important on any diet to have healthy snacks around that keep you on track, or in this case, in ketosis. Whether it's an appetizer before a meal or the 4:00 p.m. hunger games, a small bite might be the perfect way to get your ratios where you need them to be. If you're in need of a protein boost, the Smoky Maple Jerky or Greek Yogurt Deviled Eggs will do the trick. Missing that afternoon latte run? Then try the Lightened-Up Mocha Latte. Or if you're a sucker for something sweet to get you through your workday, then try our fat bombs such as the Peanut Butter or Coconut Lime Cheesecake Bombs. Whether salty or sweet, there's something for any craving, morning, noon, or night.

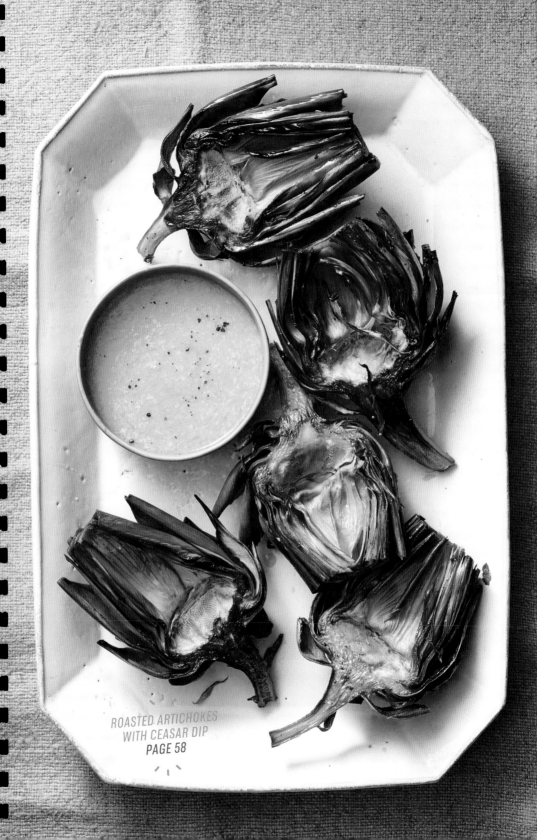

ROASTED ARTICHOKES
WITH CEASAR DIP
PAGE 58

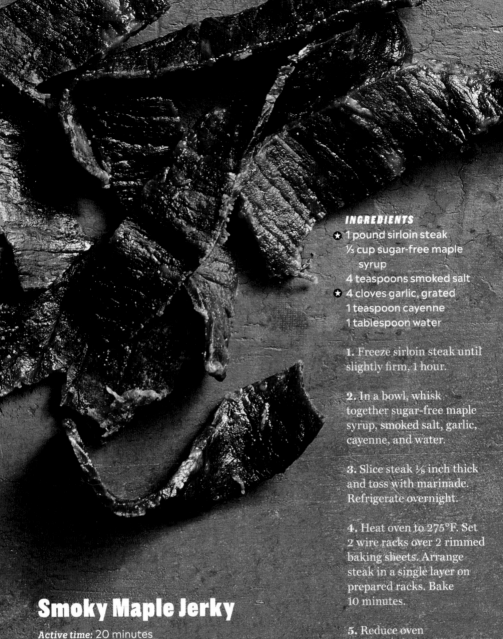

INGREDIENTS

★ 1 pound sirloin steak
⅓ cup sugar-free maple syrup
4 teaspoons smoked salt
★ 4 cloves garlic, grated
1 teaspoon cayenne
1 tablespoon water

1. Freeze sirloin steak until slightly firm, 1 hour.

2. In a bowl, whisk together sugar-free maple syrup, smoked salt, garlic, cayenne, and water.

3. Slice steak ⅛ inch thick and toss with marinade. Refrigerate overnight.

4. Heat oven to 275°F. Set 2 wire racks over 2 rimmed baking sheets. Arrange steak in a single layer on prepared racks. Bake 10 minutes.

5. Reduce oven temperature to its lowest setting, between 175°F and 200°F, and bake until steak is completely dry but still pliable, 3 to 3½ hours.

PER SERVING: 115 calories, 2 g fat (1 g saturated fat), 12 g protein, 915 mg sodium, 12 g carbohydrates, 10.5 g sugars (10.5 g added sugars), 0 g fiber

Smoky Maple Jerky

Active time: 20 minutes
Total time: 20 minutes plus marinating and baking
Makes: 8 servings

→ While on the keto diet, it's best to use grass-fed beef. Grass-fed beef is just what it sounds like: The animal consumed grass during its lifetime rather than grains. As a result, the meat has heart-healthy qualities like higher levels of omega-3s, conjugated linoleic acid, and antioxidants.

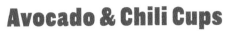

Avocado & Chili Cups

Active time: 15 minutes
Total time: 40 minutes
Makes: 8 servings

→ Garlic and onions almost always serve as a base to any sort of chili. Good thing they are two of our keto all-stars! Garlic contains a phytochemical called allicin, which fights infection and may decrease high blood pressure. Garlic's cousin, the onion, is known for its high polyphenol and flavonoid content, which reduces the risk for cancer as well as oxidative stress. See photo page 28.

INGREDIENTS

1 tablespoon olive oil
✪ 1 small onion, diced
1 small jalapeño, seeded and minced
✪ 1 clove garlic, minced
4 teaspoons chile powder
1 teaspoon ground cumin
1 14-ounce can diced green chiles, drained
✪ 1 14-ounce can diced tomatoes
Salt and pepper
✪ 1 pound ground beef
✪ 4 avocados
Crumbled Cotija cheese, cilantro leaves, diced avocado, for topping
Lime wedges, for serving

1. In a saucepan, heat olive oil on medium. Add onion, and sauté until soft, about 5 minutes. Add the jalapeño and garlic and cook for an additional minute. In the same saucepan, add beef and cook until browned, about 5 to 6 minutes. Add chile powder, cumin, chiles, tomatoes, and ¾ cup water. Season to taste with salt and pepper; cook 20 minutes.

2. Halve avocados and scoop out ⅓ of the flesh from each half around the pit's indentation. Dice scooped flesh and set aside. Fill each half with chile and top with cheese, cilantro, and diced avocado. Serve with lime wedges.

PER SERVING: 337 calories, 26 g fat (6 g saturated fat), 14 g protein, 352 mg sodium, 14 g carbohydrates, 3 g sugars (0 g added sugars), 8 g fiber

Tip
Be sure to use fresh garlic rather than bottled or jarred in recipes for higher nutrient content. Crush the garlic up to 30 minutes before cooking to initiate the formation of allicin and other healthy sulfur compounds—this process will preserve these compounds once they are heated.

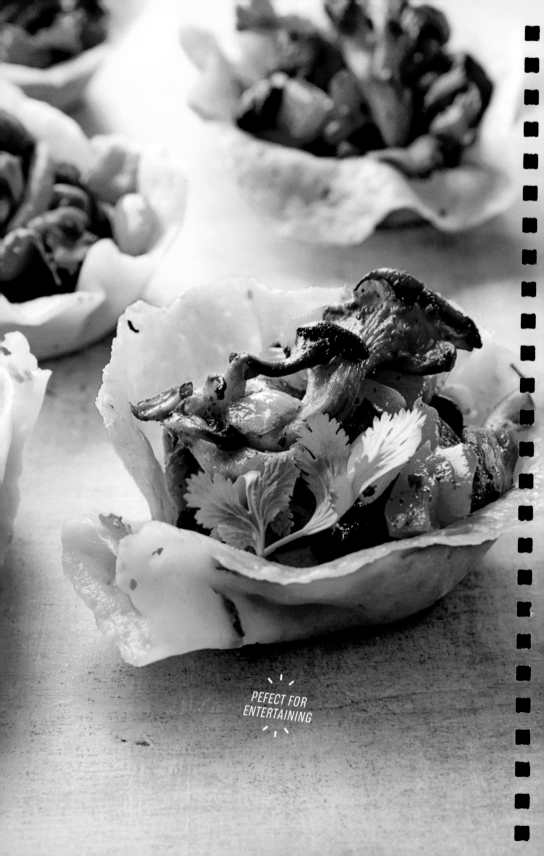

PEFECT FOR
ENTERTAINING

Veggie & Cheese Taco Cups

Active time: 10 minutes
Total time: 45 minutes plus cooling
Makes: 8 servings

➜ Mushrooms are a great substitute for meat in these taco cups. They are full of fiber, keeping you feeling full, as well as vitamins, minerals, and antioxidants. B vitamins help the body harvest energy and minerals such as selenium that aid in liver function.

INGREDIENTS

8 slices pepper jack or Colby jack cheese
✪ 1 teaspoon olive oil
½ cup chopped red bell pepper
½ cup chopped yellow bell pepper
✪ ½ cup chopped white onion
✪ 1 clove garlic, minced
✪ 8 ounces mixed mushrooms, chopped
1 teaspoon chile powder
½ teaspoon ground cumin
Salt

¼ cup chopped cilantro, for topping
4 tablespoons chopped pickled jalapeños, for topping
Lime wedges, for serving

1. Heat oven to 375°F. Place cheese slices on a parchment-lined rimmed baking sheet. Bake until bubbly, about 5 minutes. Remove from oven and let cool slightly, about 5 minutes. Gently push slices into separate muffin tin cups and let cool completely.

2. Heat olive oil in a large skillet on medium until shimmering. Add bell peppers, onion, and garlic and cook, stirring, until onion is translucent, about 5 minutes.

3. Stir in mushrooms and cook until liquid has evaporated and mushrooms are golden brown, 10 minutes. Stir in chile powder, cumin, and a pinch of salt.

4. Divide mixture among cheese cups. Top with cilantro and jalapeños. Serve with lime wedges.

PER SERVING: 117 calories, 8 g fat (5 g saturated fat), 6 g protein, 224 mg sodium, 5 g carbohydrates, 1.5 g sugars (0 g added sugars), 1 g fiber

Tip Did you know that chile powder contains both vitamins A and C? Both essential elements are great for your eye health and for fighting off infections!

Cauliflower Popcorn

Active time: 10 minutes
Total time: 40 minutes
Makes: 6 servings

➜ Cauliflower! Another one of the extremely popular low-carb substitutes that, of course, is keto-friendly. This movie munchie has blockbuster health benefits: loads of immune-boosting vitamin C, potassium, cancer-fighting phytonutrients, and 2 grams of fiber per cup. Plus, just one cup of cauliflower contains 10 percent of your daily fiber needs, which helps to keep your gut content and reduce inflammation.

INGREDIENTS

8 cups small cauliflower florets (about 1 ¼ pounds), stems trimmed
✪ 3 tablespoons olive oil
✪ ¼ cup grated Parmesan
1 teaspoon garlic powder
½ teaspoon ground turmeric
½ teaspoon kosher salt

1. Heat oven to 475°F.

2. On a large rimmed baking sheet, toss cauliflower florets with olive oil, Parmesan, garlic powder, turmeric, and salt. Roast until browned and tender, 25 to 30 minutes. Serve immediately.

PER SERVING: About 110 calories, 8 g fat (2 g saturated fat), 4 g protein, 267 mg sodium, 8 g carbohydrates, 2.5 g sugars (0 g added sugars), 3 g fiber

VARIATIONS

TRUFFLE

Omit the Parmesan, garlic powder, and turmeric. Toss the roasted cauliflower with 2 tablespoons truffle butter and ½ teaspoon ground black pepper before serving.

PER SERVING: About 120 calories, 10 g fat (3 g sat), 2 g protein, 189 mg sodium, 5 g carbohydrates, 2.5 g sugars (0 g added sugars, 2 g fiber

CHILE LIME

Substitute 1 teaspoon chile powder for the Parmesan and turmeric. Grate the zest of 1 lime over the roasted cauliflower before serving.

PER SERVING: About 90 calories, 7 g fat (1 g saturated fat), 2 g protein, 204 mg sodium, 5 g carbohydrates, 2.5 g sugars (0 g added sugars), 2 g fiber

Tip Turmeric has become famed in recent years for its anti-inflammatory properties thanks to a compound called curcumin. Reducing inflammation is key to repairing the body and fighting off pathogens. Curcumin is also important in brain function because it raises the levels of growth hormones that help to connect and increase the number of neurons in the brain.

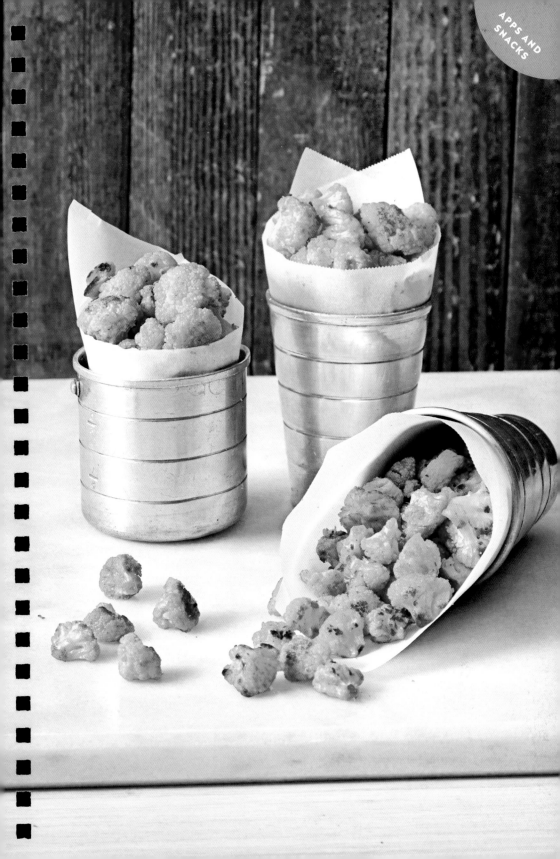

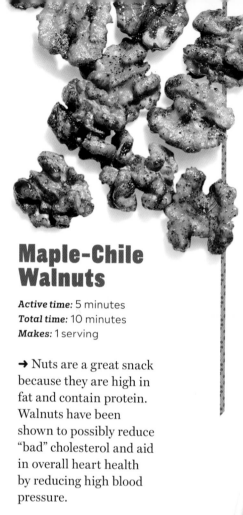

Maple-Chile Walnuts

Active time: 5 minutes
Total time: 10 minutes
Makes: 1 serving

→ Nuts are a great snack because they are high in fat and contain protein. Walnuts have been shown to possibly reduce "bad" cholesterol and aid in overall heart health by reducing high blood pressure.

INGREDIENTS

2 teaspoons sugar-free
　　maple syrup
¼ teaspoon chile powder
Sea salt
✪ 12 walnut halves

Warm maple syrup, chile powder, and a generous pinch of sea salt in a small skillet on low heat. Add walnut halves. Toss to coat. Heat 1 to 2 minutes longer. Let cool before serving.

PER SERVING: 165 calories,
16 g fat (1.5 g saturated fat),
4 g protein, 215 mg sodium,
5 g carbohydrates, 1 g sugars
(0 g added sugars), 2 g fiber

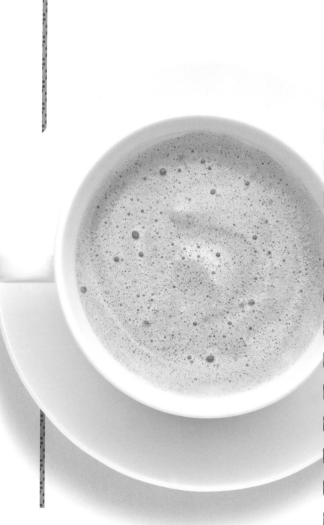

Lightened-Up Mocha Latte

Active time: 5 minutes
Total time: 5 minutes
Makes: 1 serving

→ We all love a sweet coffee drink from time to time, and even more so when it is made with chocolate. Be sure to use a low-carb, high-cacao chocolate or a stevia-sweetened chocolate, such as Lily's Sweets 70 percent Extra Dark Chocolate.

INGREDIENTS

- ✪ ¼ cup unsweetened almond or cashew milk
- 1 ounce unsweetened dark chocolate, chopped
- 2 1-ounce shots espresso or dark brewed coffee

Pour unsweetened almond or cashew milk into a glass jar. Cover and shake vigorously for 15 seconds, then remove lid and microwave on high until nice and frothy, about 30 seconds. Add chopped dark chocolate to a coffee cup, pour in 2 shots espresso or dark brewed coffee, and stir to melt chocolate. Top with milk.

PER SERVING: 185 calories, 13 g fat (7 g saturated fat), 3 g protein, 60 mg sodium, 14 g carbohydrates, 1 g sugars (0 g added sugars), 3 g fiber

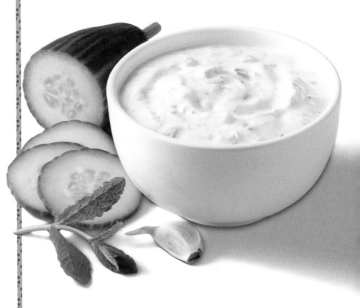

Tzatziki with Crudités

Active time: 5 minutes
Total time: 5 minutes
Makes: 1 serving

→ Dehydration is important to avoid when on the keto diet. Cucumbers are an excellent way of obtaining additional water. One cucumber is made up of about 96 percent water!

INGREDIENTS

- ✪ ⅓ cup plain yogurt
- 1 tablespoon sour cream
- ¼ cup coarsely grated cucumber
- ✪ ½ teaspoon lemon juice
- ✪ ¼ teaspoon minced garlic
- Crudités of your choice, for serving

Whisk together yogurt, sour cream, cucumber, lemon juice, and garlic. Serve with presliced veggies of your choice.

PER SERVING (DIP ONLY): 79 calories, 5 g fat (3 g saturated fat), 3 g protein, 42 mg sodium, 5 g carbohydrates, 5 g sugars (0 g added sugars), 0 g fiber

Tip **Be sure to use an English or Persian cucumber in this recipe. They are easy to grate since they have few if any seeds.**

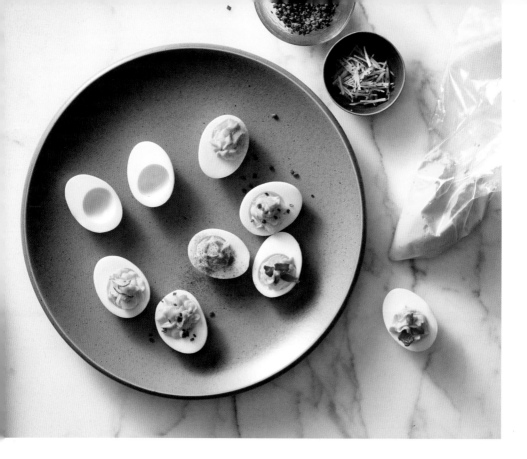

Greek Yogurt Deviled Egg

Active time: 5 minutes
Total time: 5 minutes
Makes: 12 serving

➜ It's no wonder that Greek yogurt has become the substitute for everything creamy in health-conscious recipes these days. It's high in nutrients like protein, calcium, and probiotics. Probiotics are healthy bacteria that keep your immune system and gut in check. It's important to have good bacteria living in your intestines to keep your microbiome happy.

INGREDIENTS
- ✪ 12 hard-boiled eggs
- ✪ ¾ cup Fage Total 2% Greek Yogurt
- ✪ 2 tablespoons Dijon mustard
- Sea salt
- ✪ Sliced scallions, sliced radishes, or paprika for topping

Halve each of the hard-boiled eggs. Remove yolks and mash with Greek yogurt, mustard, and sea salt to taste. Spoon into egg halves. Top with sliced scallions.

PER SERVING: 90 calories, 6 g fat (2 g saturated fat), 8 g protein, 166 mg sodium, 1 g carbohydrates, 1 g sugars (0 g added sugars), 0 g fiber

WHAT ARE PROBIOTICS?

Probiotics, the good bacteria that help keep our gut healthy, have gotten a ton of well-deserved attention over the past few years. Prevalent in yogurt, probiotics may seem strange as a daily supplement. But having an abundance of this good bacteria helps fight off sickness and strengthen your immune system. With more positive research, probiotics are being recommended by disease specialists to prevent digestive diseases that cannot be treated with standard medical practices.

Since there are so many types of good bacteria, probiotics can also be used to treat or maintain several gut concerns. Probiotics have been found to possibly help with a negative side effect of the keto diet, constipation. It's important to note that you should still consult a doctor before taking these supplements as they do not have the same testing and approval process as standard drugs.

Prosciutto Scallion Bundles

Total time: 20 minutes
Makes: 8 servings

→ Also called green onions, scallions are a pungent relative of onions, leeks, shallots, and chives. The green part has a mild onion flavor while the white parts carry more bite. Wrapped in prosciutto, this onion variety packs fiber with few calories and makes a great appetizer or even a side!

INGREDIENTS
- ✪ 24 scallions, trimmed
  Kosher salt and pepper
  4 thin slices prosciutto, halved lengthwise
- ✪ 2 tablespoons olive oil

1. Season scallions with ¼ teaspoon each salt and pepper. Wrap 1 piece prosciutto around 3 scallions (white and light green parts), pressing lightly to adhere. Repeat with remaining prosciutto and scallions to make 8 bundles.

2. Heat oil in a large skillet on medium-high. Working in 2 batches, cook scallion bundles, turning occasionally, until browned and crisp on all sides, 3 to 4 minutes, adding more oil to skillet as necessary. Transfer to paper towels, then a platter to serve.

PER SERVING: 60 calories, 4.5 g fat (1 g saturated fat), 3 g protein, 230 mg sodium, 3 g carbohydrates, 0 g sugars (0 g added sugars), 1 g fiber

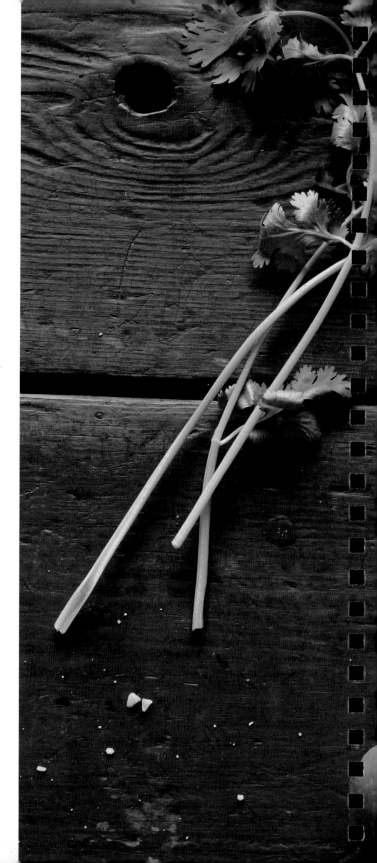

Go-To Guacamole

Active time: 10 minutes
Total time: 10 minutes
Makes: 4 servings

➜ Fresh herbs are a flavor enhancer for any recipe, but did you know they also have some amazing health benefits? Cilantro is an ancient herb with a robust, savory flavor. It is also a great source of antioxidants, helps cleanse our bloodstream of toxins, lowers blood sugar, and reduces inflammation.

INGREDIENTS

- ✪ 2 avocados, chopped
- ✪ ½ small Roman tomato, diced
- ¼ cup chopped cilantro
- ¼ small onion, diced
- ½ small jalapeño, minced
- ✪ 1 clove garlic, minced
- ✪ 2 tablespoons fresh lime juice
- Salt and pepper

In a bowl, combine avocados, tomato, cilantro, onion, jalapeño, garlic, and lime juice. Mix to desired consistency and season to taste with salt and pepper.

PER SERVING: 168 calories, 4.5 g fat (2 g saturated fat), 2 g protein, 154 mg sodium, 10 g carbohydrates, 1 g sugars (0 g added sugars), 7 g fiber

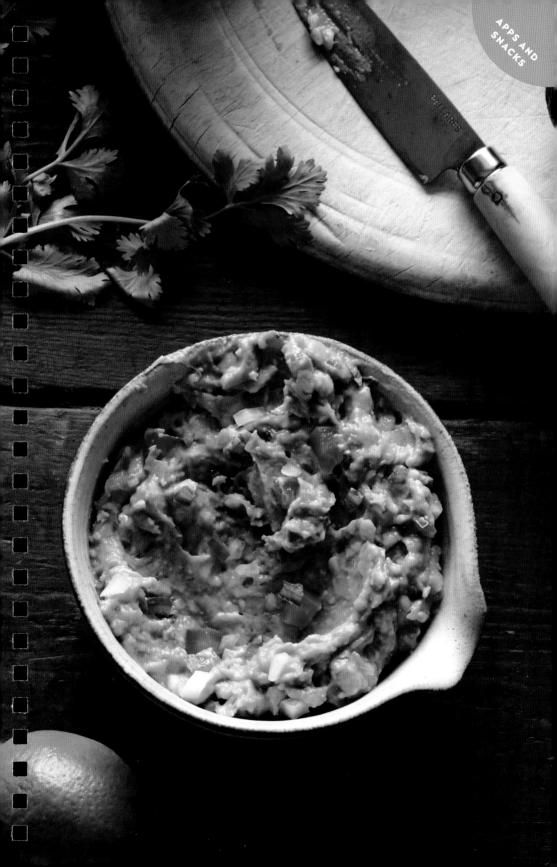

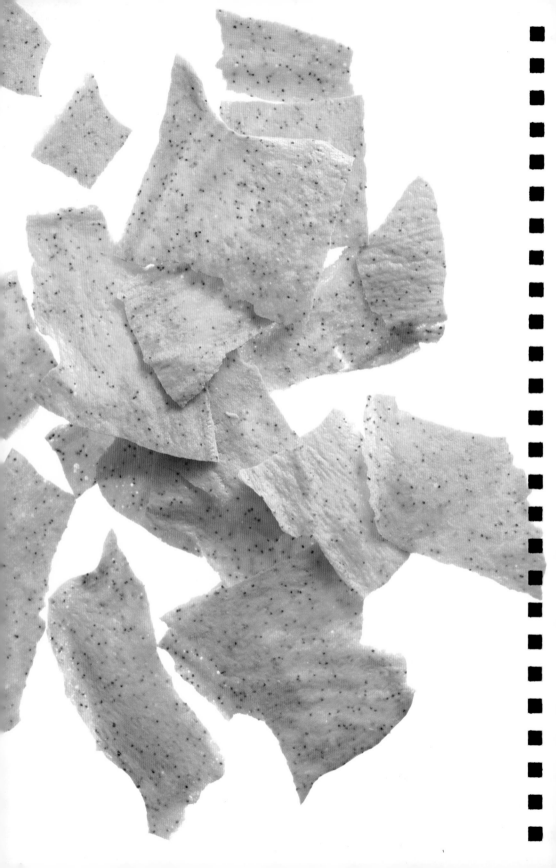

Poppy Seed–Cheddar Bark

Active time: 10 minutes plus 20 minutes freezing
Total time: 1 hour 20 minutes
Makes: 8 servings

→ Who doesn't love a crunchy, cheesy snack? The salty flavor can satisfy any afternoon craving. This recipe is packed with a protein combo of cheese and egg whites to keep you fueled throughout the afternoon. Plus, 1 teaspoon of poppy seeds contains enough calcium and phosphorus to meet 4 percent of your daily needs, 2 to 4 percent of your daily needs for iron, and 2 to 3 percent of your daily zinc—wow!

INGREDIENTS
8 ounces extra-sharp Cheddar, coarsely grated
✪ 3 large egg whites
½ cup almond flour
✪ 2 teaspoons poppy seeds

1. In a food processor, pulse Cheddar and egg whites until smooth. Add almond flour and poppy seeds; pulse to combine.

2. Divide mixture (it will be sticky) between 2 large pieces of parchment paper cut to the size of a baking sheet. Cover each piece with another piece of parchment and roll out mixture between the layers until paper-thin.

3. Transfer the parchment and dough to 2 baking sheets and freeze until firm, 20 minutes.

4. Meanwhile, heat oven to 300°F.

5. Discard the top layers of parchment and bake, rotating sheets halfway through cooking, until mixture is golden brown and crisp, 45 to 50 minutes.

6. Let cool, then break bark into pieces.

PER SERVING: 162 calories, 13 g fat (6 g saturated fat), 10 g protein, 203 mg sodium, 3 g carbohydrates, 0 g sugars (0 g added sugars), 1 g fiber

Tip Try topping with other seeds or even using a combination of seeds in this recipe as well. Keto-friendly seeds include chia seeds, flaxseed, hemp seeds, sesame seeds, and sunflower seeds.

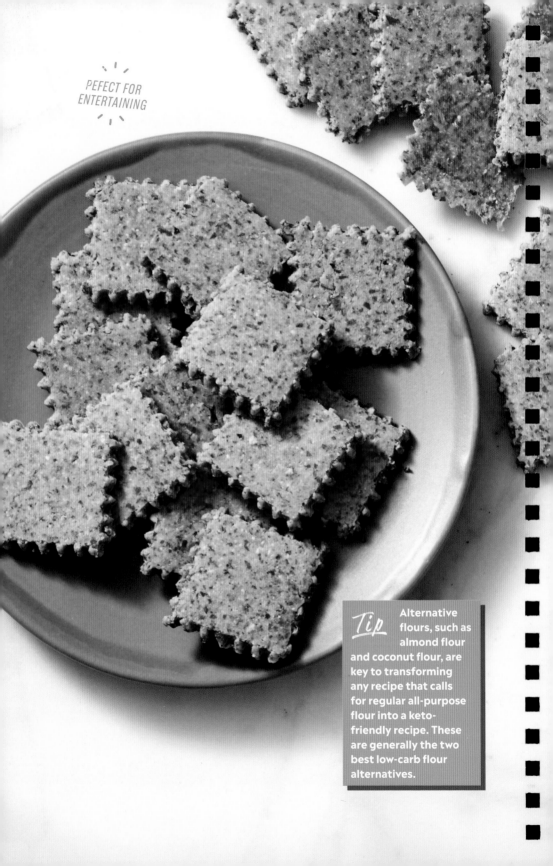

PEFECT FOR
ENTERTAINING

Tip Alternative flours, such as almond flour and coconut flour, are key to transforming any recipe that calls for regular all-purpose flour into a keto-friendly recipe. These are generally the two best low-carb flour alternatives.

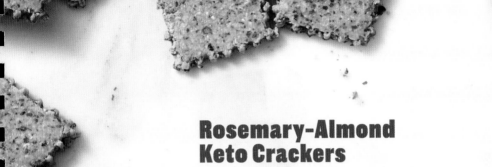

Rosemary-Almond Keto Crackers

Active time: 20 minutes
Total time: 1 hour
Makes: 14 servings (10 1-inch square crackers)

→ With just a couple of ingredient swaps, crackers can become keto-friendly instantly. Flaxseed meal is one swap worth making—1 tablespoon contains 2 grams of polyunsaturated fatty acids (including omega-3s) and 2 grams of dietary fiber, essential nutrients the average cracker usually does not provide.

INGREDIENTS

- ✪ 2 ½ cups almond flour
- ½ cup coconut flour
- 1 teaspoon ground flaxseed meal
- ½ teaspoon dried rosemary, crumbled
- ½ teaspoon onion powder
- ¼ teaspoon kosher salt
- ✪ 3 large eggs
- ✪ 1 tablespoon olive oil

1. Heat oven to 325°F. Line a baking sheet with parchment paper.

2. In a large bowl, whisk together flours, flaxseed meal, rosemary, onion powder, and salt. Add eggs and olive oil and mix to combine. Continue mixing until dough forms a large ball, about 1 minute.

3. Sandwich dough between 2 pieces of parchment and roll to ¼ inch thick. Cut into squares and place on prepared sheet. Bake until crackers are golden brown, 12 to 15 minutes. Let cool.

PER SERVING: 160 calories, 13 g fat (2 g saturated fat), 6 g protein, 60 mg sodium, 7 g carbohydrates, 1 g sugars (0 g added sugars), 4 g fiber

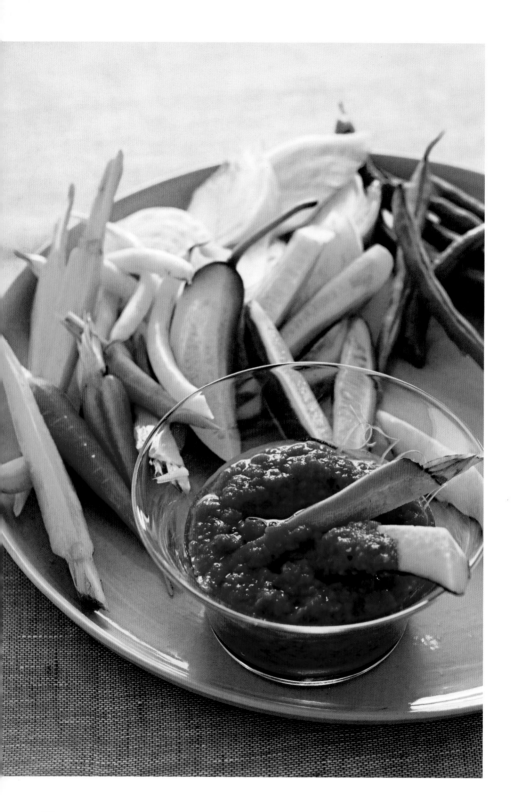

Crudités with Romesco Sauce

Active time: 20 minutes
Total time: 35 minutes plus chilling
Makes: 8 servings

→ Romesco sauce hails from Spain and is made from red bell peppers and almonds. This nibbling platter is packed with beta-carotene and vitamin C, two cancer-fighting antioxidants that work together to ward off cellular damage. Red bell pepper and tomatoes—the base of the tangy sauce—are also a good source of cancer-protective lycopene.

INGREDIENTS

3 large red bell peppers
✪ 3 tablespoons extra-virgin olive oil
✪ ¼ cup sliced almonds
✪ 2 cloves garlic, smashed
1 plum tomato, quartered
1 tablespoon red wine vinegar
1 teaspoon paprika
¾ teaspoon salt
¼ teaspoon freshly ground black pepper
4 carrots, trimmed and cut into 2-inch strips, for serving
1 large or 2 small cucumbers, cut into 2-inch strips, for serving
1 bulb fennel, trimmed and cut into 2-inch strips, for serving
½ pound yellow wax beans, trimmed, for serving
½ pound green beans, trimmed, for serving

1. Heat broiler with the rack placed about 4 inches from the heat source.

2. Place whole red peppers on a rimmed baking sheet and broil, turning every 3 minutes, until skins are blistered and charred, 12 to 15 minutes. Transfer peppers to a medium bowl, cover with plastic wrap, and let steam 10 minutes. Peel, and discard stems, seeds, and ribs.

3. Meanwhile, while peppers roast, combine olive oil, almonds, and garlic in a small skillet on medium heat. Cook, stirring often, until almonds and garlic are lightly golden, 4 to 5 minutes. Remove from heat.

4. Put roasted peppers and tomato in a blender and puree. Add olive oil mixture and puree. Add vinegar, paprika, salt, and black pepper and puree. Transfer to a serving bowl and chill sauce 20 minutes or until ready to serve.

5. Arrange carrots, cucumber, fennel, and beans on a platter. Serve with romesco sauce.

PER SERVING: 124 calories, 7 g fat (1 g saturated fat), 3 g protein, 222 mg sodium, 15 g carbohydrates, 8 g sugars (0 g added sugars), 4 g fiber

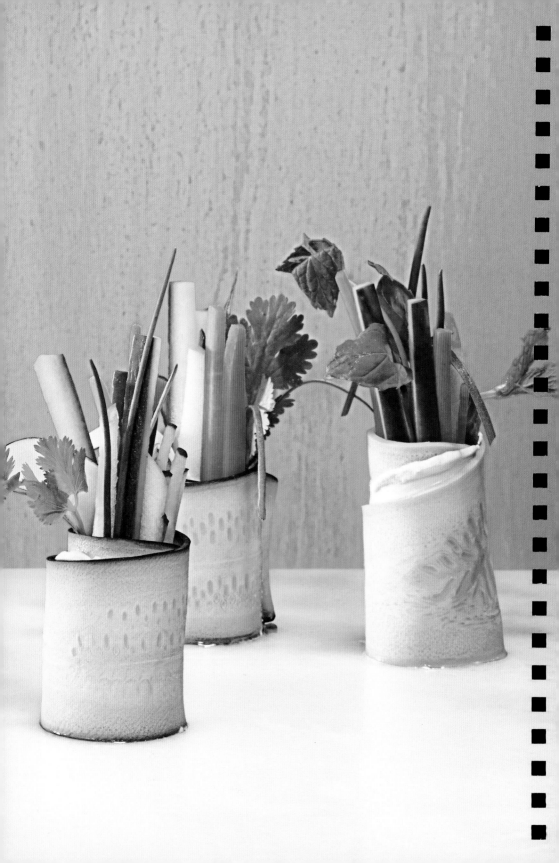

Veggie Rolls

Active time: 10 minutes
Total time: 10 minutes
Makes: 8 serving

→ Finding carb substitutes for noodles or wraps can be challenging. Zucchini serves as the perfect low-carb option in this recipe, and also provides vitamins A and C, antioxidants, and fiber. Wrapping it around a filling that's high in fat, like cream cheese, helps you to happily maintain ketosis.

INGREDIENTS

4 zucchini or yellow squash
8 ounces cream cheese, softened
⅛ teaspoon salt
Flavorings, veggies, and/or fruits

1. With a vegetable peeler, peel squash into wide ribbons.

2. Mix cream cheese and salt with flavorings.

3. Cut vegetables and fruits into 2-inch-long matchsticks. Spread 1 tablespoon flavored cream cheese on one end of a veggie ribbon. Add veggie and fruit matchsticks and roll each tightly into a bundle. Make up to 1 hour ahead; let stand at room temperature.

VARIATIONS

RED PEPPER-BASIL

Mix ½ cup roasted red peppers, finely chopped, into cream cheese. Roll with basil leaves, bell peppers, and green apples.

PER SERVING: 168 calories, 10 g fat (6 g saturated fat), 4 g protein, 249 mg sodium, 16 g carbohydrates, 8 g sugars (0 g added sugars), 5 g fiber

ASIAN GARDEN

Mix 1 tablespoon soy sauce and 2 teaspoons fresh lime juice into the cream cheese. Roll with radishes, scallions, and carrots.

PER SERVING: 129 calories, 10 g fat (6 g saturated fat), 4 g protein, 576 mg sodium, 7 g carbohydrates, 4.5 g sugars (0 g added sugars), 3 g fiber

VEGGIE CHILI

Mix ½ cup coarsely grated Cheddar and 1 teaspoon chile powder into cream cheese. Roll with cilantro, cucumber, and jicama.

PER SERVING: 243 calories, 19.5 g fat (11 g saturated fat), 10 g protein, 351 mg sodium, 8 g carbohydrates, 4 g sugars (0 g added sugars), 3 g fiber

ZIPPY PEAR

Mix 1½ tablespoons bottled horseradish and 1 tablespoon snipped fresh chives into cream cheese. Roll with parsley, pears, and celery.

PER SERVING: 177 calories, 10 g fat (6 g saturated fat), 4 g protein, 188 mg sodium, 10 g carbohydrates, 6 g sugars (0 g added sugars), 3 g fiber

Roasted Artichokes with Caesar Dip

Active time: 45 minutes
Total time: 1 hour 20 minutes
Makes: 6 servings

→ Artichokes are low in fat and high in fiber and rank among the most antioxidant-rich of all vegetables. Served with a buttery and flavorful dipping sauce, this keto-friendly vegetable is a perfect appetizer for your next gathering.

INGREDIENTS

- 3 globe artichokes
- ✪ 2 lemons
- ✪ 4 tablespoons olive oil
  Kosher salt
- ✪ 1 small clove garlic, pressed
  1 teaspoon Dijon mustard
  ½ teaspoon Worcestershire sauce
  ¼ cup grated Parmesan

1. Heat oven to 425°F and line a rimmed baking sheet with foil.

2. Rinse and dry artichokes with a paper towel. Trim stems and cut ¼-inch off each top. Use kitchen shears to cut off tip of each leaf. Use hands to pull and loosen leaves to open up artichokes. Slice artichokes in half vertically and use a small knife to cut out fuzzy centers and purple leaves.

3. Place artichoke halves on the baking sheet, squeeze juice of half of 1 lemon on cut sides, and rub lemon half over each. Drizzle with 1 tablespoon olive oil and season with ¼ teaspoon salt. Flip artichokes and repeat with other lemon half, 1 tablespoon olive oil, and ¼ teaspoon salt.

4. Arrange artichokes cut sides down, cover with foil and roast until golden brown and tender, 35 to 40 minutes.

5. Meanwhile, sprinkle ¼ teaspoon salt over garlic; using a large knife, rub and scrape salt into garlic to make paste. Transfer to a bowl.

6. Finely grate zest of remaining lemon into the bowl, then squeeze in juice (you should have at least 3 tablespoons). Whisk in mustard, Worcestershire sauce, and remaining 2 tablespoons oil. Stir in Parmesan. Serve with artichokes for dipping.

PER SERVING: 155 calories, 12 g fat (2 g saturated fat), 4 g protein, 300 mg sodium, 9 g carb, 4 g fiber, 1 g sugars (0 g added sugars)

Sesame–Smoked Salmon Bombs

Active time: 10 minutes
Total time: 10 minutes plus chilling
Makes: 12 servings

→ The rich flavor and buttery texture of smoked salmon can make any dish even more decadent. Salmon is also a rich source of vitamin D as well as omega-3s. Omega-3s and the healthy fats found in salmon and other seafood can aid in weight loss, prevent heart disease, and even boost your mood!

INGREDIENTS

4 ounces cream cheese, at room temperature
¼ cup butter, at room temperature
✪ ½ teaspoon grated lemon zest
✪ 2 teaspoons fresh lemon juice
1 teaspoon toasted sesame oil
½ teaspoon ground ginger
✪ 2 ounces smoked salmon, chopped
3 tablespoons sesame seeds or chopped pistachios

1. Line a rimmed baking sheet with parchment paper and set aside. In a medium bowl, stir together cream cheese, butter, lemon zest, lemon juice, sesame oil, and ginger until very well blended. Stir in smoked salmon until combined.

2. Drop a tablespoon of the mixture on the prepared baking sheet and repeat until you have 12 equal-size mounds.

3. Place the baking sheet in the refrigerator and chill until bombs are firm, 1½ to 2 hours.

4. Place sesame seeds or nuts in a small, shallow dish. Using your hands, quickly shape the bombs into balls and toss them in sesame seeds to coat. Store in a sealed container in the refrigerator for up to 1 week.

PER SERVING: 85 calories, 9 g fat (5 g saturated fat), 2 g protein, 93 mg sodium, 1 g carbohydrates, 0 g sugars (0 g added sugars), 0 g fiber

Peanut Butter Bombs

Active time: 15 minutes
Total time: 15 minutes plus chilling
Makes: 12 servings

➔ Because it excludes sugar, the keto diet can make it seem like sweet treats are not an option. Luckily, there is a fix! Use liquid stevia or erythritol to make even the most decadent treats low-carb. Be careful when using stevia since it is 200 to 300 times sweeter than regular sugar.

INGREDIENTS

4 ounces cream cheese, at room temperature
✪ ½ cup natural peanut butter
2 tablespoons softened coconut oil
12 drops liquid stevia
⅛ teaspoon ground cinnamon
⅓ cup sugar-free dark chocolate chips
½ cup unsalted peanuts, chopped

1. Line a rimmed baking sheet with parchment paper and set aside.

2. In a medium bowl, stir together cream cheese, peanut butter, coconut oil, stevia, and cinnamon until well blended. Stir in chocolate chips.

3. Drop a tablespoon of the mixture on the prepared baking sheet and repeat until you have 12 equal-size mounds.

4. Place the baking sheet in the refrigerator and chill until bombs are firm, about 1½ hours.

5. Place chopped peanuts in a small, shallow dish. Using your hands, shape the bombs into balls and roll them in chopped peanuts to coat. Store in a sealed container in the refrigerator up to 1 week.

PER SERVING: 180 calories, 15 g fat (6 g saturated fat), 5 g protein, 66 mg sodium, 7 g carbohydrates, 1 g sugars (0 g added sugars), 2 g fiber

---

Chocolate Pudding Bombs

Active time: 10 minutes
Total time: 10 minutes plus chilling
Makes: 12 servings

➔ Coconut oil has been praised for its abundance of healthy saturated fats. These fats can quickly be converted into a great source of energy and aid in weight loss—especially on keto!

INGREDIENTS

¼ cup coconut oil
¼ cup unsweetened cocoa
1 teaspoon instant espresso-coffee powder
✪ ½ cup cashew butter
2 ounces cream cheese, at room temperature
12 drops liquid stevia

1. Line a rimmed baking sheet with parchment paper and set aside.

2. In a medium bowl, microwave coconut oil on High until melted, about 30 seconds. Whisk in cocoa and espresso powder, cashew butter, cream cheese, and stevia until smooth and well blended.

3. Drop a tablespoon of the mixture on the prepared baking sheet and repeat until you have 12 equal-size mounds.

4. Place the baking sheet in the refrigerator and chill until bombs are firm, about 30 minutes.

5. Store in a sealed container in the refrigerator for up to 1 week.

PER SERVING: 125 calories, 12 g fat (6 g saturated fat), 3 g protein, 17 mg sodium, 4 g carbohydrates, 0 g sugars (0 g added sugars), 1 g fiber

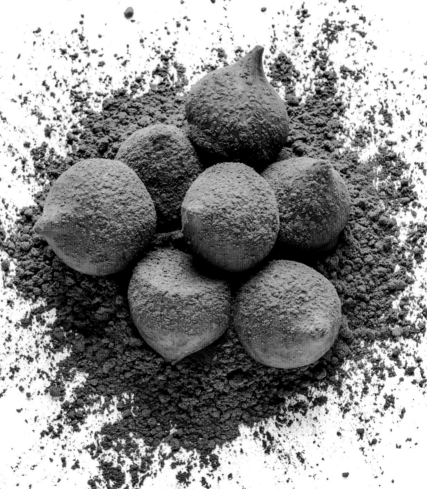

Coconut-Lime Cheesecake Bombs

Active time: 10 minutes
Total time: 10 minutes plus chilling
Makes: 12 servings

→ Here is the solution to your dessert craving. Grated unsweetened coconut is high in fiber as well as copper and manganese, the former helping fat metabolize and the latter benefiting heart health and bones. Be sure to eat coconut only occasionally since it's high in calories and moderate in carbs.

INGREDIENTS

⅔ cup softened coconut oil
6 tablespoons cream cheese, at room temperature
✪ 2 teaspoons grated lime zest
✪ 2 teaspoons fresh lime juice
8 drops liquid stevia
1 drop pure coconut extract or pure almond extract
7 tablespoons finely grated unsweetened coconut

1. Line a rimmed baking sheet with parchment paper and set aside.

2. In a medium bowl, stir together coconut oil, cream cheese, lime zest, lime juice, stevia, and extract until very well blended. Stir in 4 tablespoons grated coconut until combined.

3. Drop a tablespoon of the mixture on the prepared baking sheet and repeat until you have 12 equal-size mounds.

4. Place the baking sheet in the refrigerator and chill until bombs are firm, 1 to 2 hours.

5. Place 3 tablespoons grated coconut in a small, shallow dish. Using your hands, quickly shape the bombs into balls and toss them in coconut to coat. Store in a sealed container in the refrigerator for up to 1 week.

PER SERVING: 155 calories, 16 g fat (13 g saturated fat), 1 g protein, 24 mg sodium, 1 g carbohydrates, 0.5 g sugars (0 g added sugars), 1 g fiber

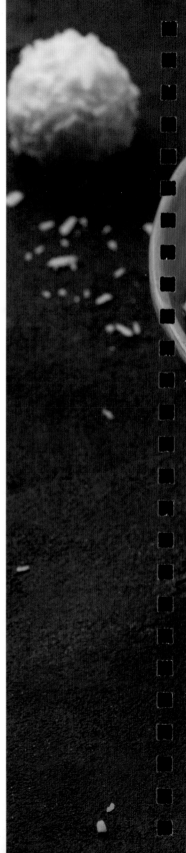

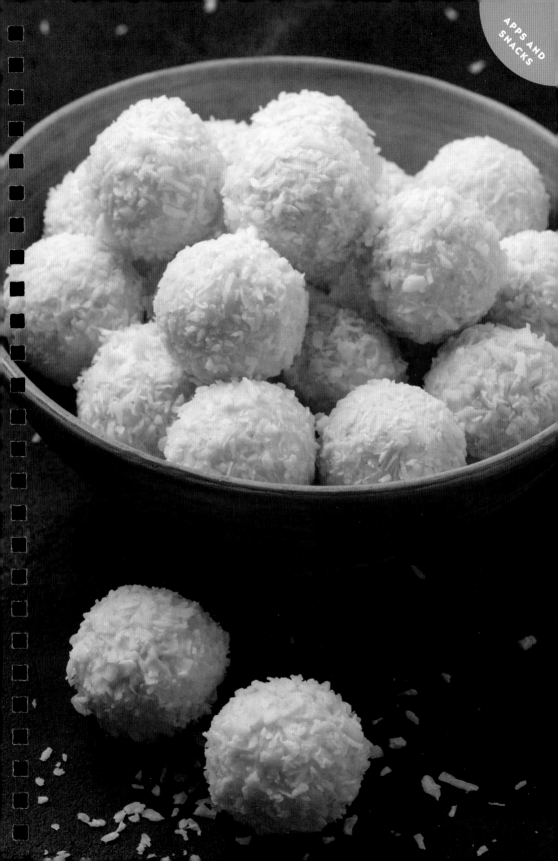

Chapter 3

Soups & Salads

Soups and salads—they are good for lunch or dinner and can stand alone or be the perfect meal combo together. Better yet, they can also be made ahead and packed for the ideal weekday lunch at the office or for an easy dinner after a long day. No matter the occasion, there is a salad or soup that will suit your mood. Try the Wild Salmon Salad or the Roasted Cauliflower "Steak" Salad for two of the more filling options. The Rainbow Chicken Slaw or the Ratatouille Salad are just right for highlighting delicious summer produce. Plus, as for soup, the Savory Tomato Soup will pair with any of these salads, while the Thai Green Curry Soup is a filling entrée that will make you forget about calling your favorite local takeout. Cool off on a hot day with a cup of the Cucumber-Raspberry Gazpacho. With these recipes in your back pocket, you will see how delicious keto soups and salads can be.

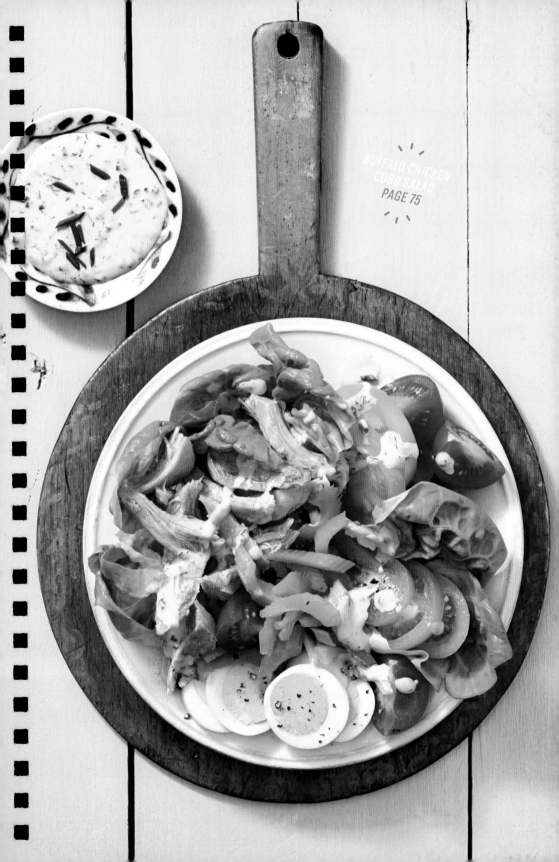

BUFFALO CHICKEN
COBB SALAD
PAGE 75

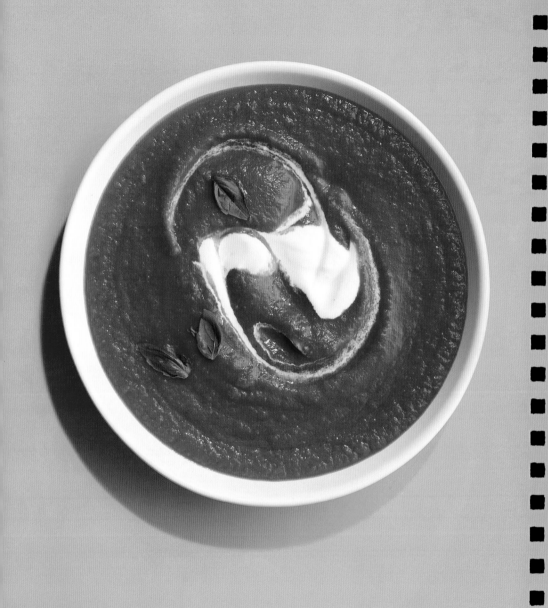

Savory Tomato Soup

Active time: 10 minutes
Total time: 40 minutes
Makes: 4 servings

→ Many store-bought tomato soups are packed with added sugar. In this easy homemade version, carrots boost vitamin A and flavor in lieu of high-fructose corn syrup.

INGREDIENTS
- ✪ 1 tablespoon olive oil
- ½ small carrot, grated
- ✪ ½ small onion, thinly sliced
- ✪ 1 tablespoon tomato paste
- ✪ 1 28-ounce can crushed tomatoes with basil
- 2 cups low-sodium vegetable or chicken broth
- Salt and pepper
- ¼ cup plain whole-milk yogurt, for topping (optional)
- Basil leaves, for topping (optional)

1. Heat olive oil in a large saucepan on medium-high. Add carrot and onion and cook, stirring occasionally, until vegetables begin to soften, about 5 minutes.

2. Add tomato paste and cook 1 minute more. Add tomatoes (with juice) and broth. Bring to a boil, then reduce heat and simmer until vegetables are tender and soup is thick, 25 minutes.

3. Process soup in a blender until smooth. Season to taste with salt and pepper. To serve, top with yogurt and sprinkle with basil, if desired.

PER SERVING: 112 calories, 3.5 g fat (0 g saturated fat), 4 g protein, 469 mg sodium, 17 g carbohydrates, 8 g sugars (0 g added sugars), 8 g fiber

Tip
Tomato paste is a secret weapon to add a punch of tangy tomato flavor to a recipe. A little bit of this concentrated paste goes a long way. Be sure to look for brands with "no salt added" on the label.

Thai Green Curry Soup

Active time: 10 minutes
Total time: 40 minutes
Makes: 4 servings

➜ Green curry paste is responsible for giving this soup its unique and delicious flavor. Turmeric, kaffir lime, ginger, chile peppers, and lemongrass all contribute to this unique paste—but also help reduce inflammation, aid in digestion, and prevent colds.

INGREDIENTS

1 pound asparagus
4 teaspoons coconut oil
✪ 1 small onion, chopped
1-inch piece fresh ginger, peeled and chopped
1 cup small cauliflower florets
1 quart reduced-sodium vegetable broth
1 13.5-ounce can light coconut milk
1 tablespoon Thai green curry paste
✪ 5 ounces fresh spinach

½ teaspoon kosher salt
½ teaspoon black pepper
1 cup snap peas, trimmed and halved
Mint leaves, for topping

1. Trim asparagus, set stalks aside, and coarsely chop ends.

2. In a pot, heat 2 teaspoons coconut oil on medium-high. Add onion, ginger, asparagus ends, and cauliflower. Cook until vegetables soften, about 5 minutes. Add broth, coconut milk, and curry paste. Bring to a boil, then reduce to a simmer and cook until vegetables are tender, 8 minutes. Add spinach and cook until spinach wilts.

3. Remove from heat, process soup in batches in a blender, and season with salt and pepper. Cut asparagus stalks into 1-inch pieces. Heat 2 teaspoons coconut oil in a skillet on medium-high. Add stalks and snap peas. Sauté until crisp-tender, about 3 minutes. Serve soup topped with veggies and mint leaves.

PER SERVING: 178 calories, 12 g fat (10 g saturated fat), 5 g protein, 575 mg sodium, 14 g carbohydrates, 5 g sugars (0 g added sugars), 4 g fiber

Tip **Ginger has become wildly popular not only for its spicy bite but for its medicinal properties. Ginger aids in warding off the common cold and nausea, and improves digestion, thanks to the anti-inflammatory compound called gingerol. Try slicing fresh ginger and adding it to hot tea—it will be a delight to your tummy all day.**

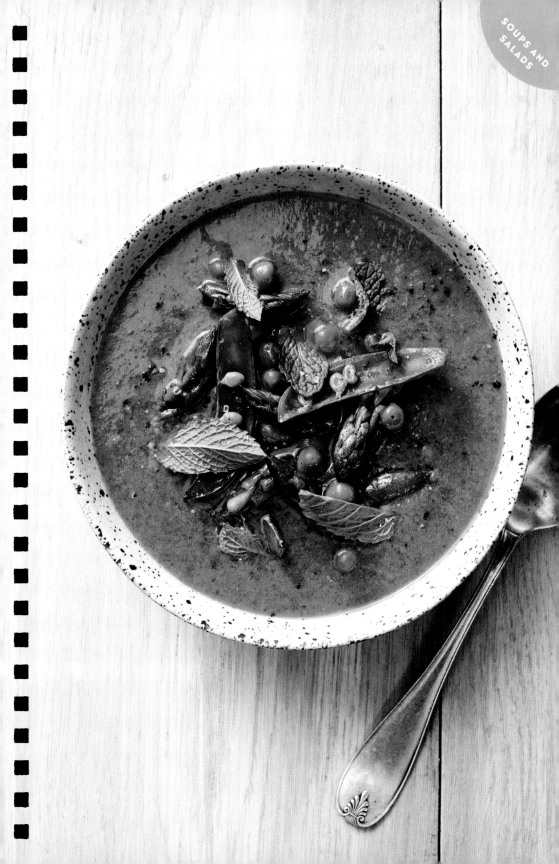

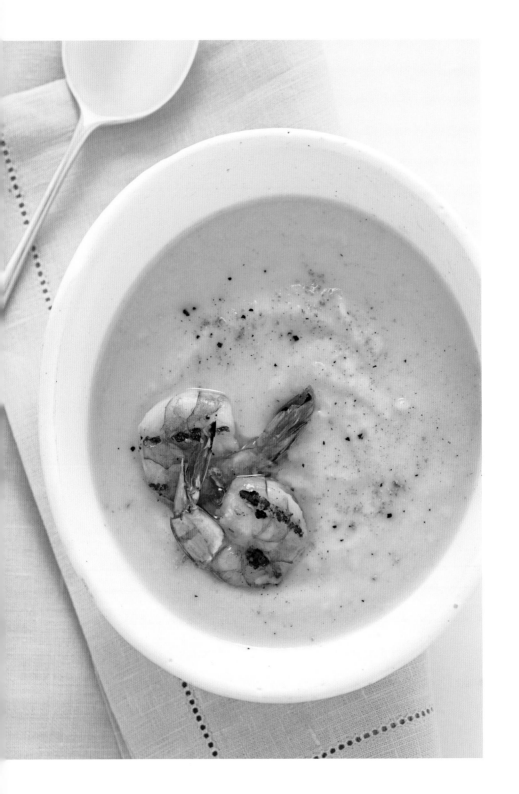

Cauliflower Soup with Grilled Shrimp

Active time: 30 minutes
Total time: 50 minutes
Makes: 4 servings

→ One cup of cauliflower contains nearly two-thirds of a full day's worth of vitamin C, a high intake of which may be linked to a lower risk of rheumatoid arthritis. This soup packs potassium, too—900 mg—almost twice the recommended daily value.

INGREDIENTS

- ✪ 3 teaspoons olive oil
- ✪ 1 cup chopped red onion (1 medium)
- ½ cup chopped celery
- 4 cups cauliflower florets (about 1½ pounds)
- ½ teaspoon ground coriander
- 2 14.5-ounce cans low-sodium chicken or vegetable broth
- ✪ 12 ounces large shrimp, peeled and deveined (8 to 12 shrimp)
- ½ teaspoon salt
- ¼ teaspoon freshly ground black pepper
- ⅓ cup fat-free evaporated milk

1. Heat a grill to medium-high. Coat the grill rack with cooking spray.

2. Heat 2 teaspoons olive oil in a soup pot on medium. Add onion and celery and cook, stirring occasionally, 6 to 7 minutes. Stir in cauliflower and coriander. Cook 2 minutes. Add broth and bring to a boil. Reduce heat to medium-low, cover, and simmer until cauliflower is tender, 20 minutes. Remove from heat and let cool 5 minutes.

3. Season shrimp with ¼ teaspoon salt, ⅛ teaspoon pepper, and 1 teaspoon olive oil. Grill until opaque, 2 to 3 minutes per side.

4. Puree soup in batches. Return to pot. Stir in milk, ¼ teaspoon salt, and ⅛ teaspoon pepper. Warm soup on medium heat until heated through, about 5 minutes. Serve with shrimp.

PER SERVING: 178 calories, 5 g fat (1 g saturated fat), 21 g protein, 429 mg sodium, 15 g carbohydrates, 7 g sugars (0 g added sugars), 3 g fiber

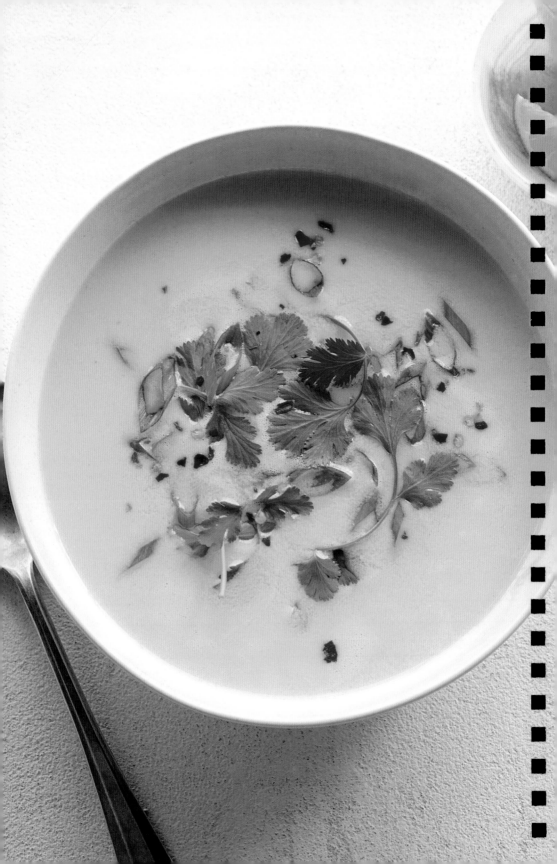

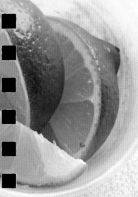

Fresh Corn & Coconut Soup

Active time: 5 minutes
Total time: 15 minutes
Makes: 4 servings

→ Sweet and creamy thanks to the corn and coconut milk, this soup may seem unhealthy. Surprise! It has several health benefits. The corn contains fiber and resistant starches that help with digestion and weight loss. The coconut milk contains MCT fats, which your body uses more rapidly for energy compared with other fats.

INGREDIENTS

1 cup corn kernels
1 13.5-ounce can full-fat coconut milk
✪ 1 lime
2 teaspoons fish sauce
½ teaspoon red pepper flakes
✪ 2 scallions, sliced, white parts only
⅛ teaspoon kosher salt
Cilantro, red pepper flakes, scallion greens, lime wedges, for serving

In a blender, combine corn kernels, coconut milk, juice of lime, fish sauce, red pepper flakes, scallions, and salt. Puree until smooth. Strain; discard solids. Serve with cilantro, red pepper flakes, scallion greens, and lime wedges.

PER SERVING: 234 calories, 21 g fat (18 g saturated fat), 4 g protein, 273 mg sodium, 13 g carbohydrates, 2 g sugars (0 g added sugars), 1 g fiber

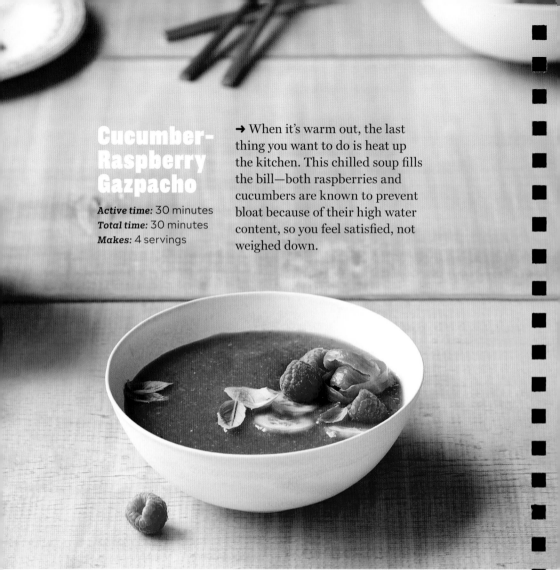

Cucumber-Raspberry Gazpacho

Active time: 30 minutes
Total time: 30 minutes
Makes: 4 servings

→ When it's warm out, the last thing you want to do is heat up the kitchen. This chilled soup fills the bill—both raspberries and cucumbers are known to prevent bloat because of their high water content, so you feel satisfied, not weighed down.

INGREDIENTS

2 cups raspberries, plus more for serving
✪ 2 medium tomatoes, seeded and chopped
1 seedless cucumber, peeled and chopped, plus more for serving
1 jalapeño, seeded and chopped

4 pickled cherry peppers (such as Peppadew)
¼ cup basil leaves, plus more for serving
✪ 3 tablespoons lemon juice
✪ 2 cloves garlic, smashed
½ teaspoon kosher salt
⅛ teaspoon ground cumin (optional)

1. In a blender, puree all ingredients until smooth. Strain through a fine-mesh sieve into a large bowl.

2. Divide among 4 chilled bowls and top with additional raspberries, cucumber, and basil.

PER SERVING: 76 calories, 1 g fat (0 g saturated fat), 2 g protein, 218 mg sodium, 17 g carbohydrates, 8 g sugars (0 g added sugars), 7 g fiber

Buffalo Chicken Cobb Salad

Active time: 35 minutes
Total time: 40 minutes
Makes: 6 servings

→ The classic wing flavors pair up with lettuce, tomatoes, and eggs and get dressed with a silky Avocado-Buttermilk Ranch Dressing. With eight different keto all-star ingredients, this salad is packed with as much nutrition as flavor.

INGREDIENTS

- 1 cup buttermilk
- ✪ 1 ripe small avocado
- ✪ 2 tablespoons fresh lemon juice
- ✪ 1 clove garlic
- ¾ teaspoon kosher salt
- ¾ teaspoon ground black pepper
- 2 tablespoons chopped fresh dill
- ✪ 1 tablespoon snipped fresh chives
- ✪ 2 cups rotisserie chicken meat cut into bite-size pieces
- ⅓ cup cayenne pepper hot sauce
- 1 teaspoon distilled white vinegar
- ✪ 6 hard-cooked eggs
- 3 stalks celery
- ✪ 3 small tomatoes
- ✪ 1 head butter lettuce or Boston lettuce

1. In a blender, puree buttermilk, avocado, lemon juice, garlic, kosher salt, and ground black pepper until smooth. Transfer to a container; stir in chopped fresh dill and snipped fresh chives. Makes 1 cup.

2. In a medium bowl, toss chicken with hot sauce and vinegar until well coated.

3. Slice eggs crosswise and thinly slice celery; cut tomatoes into wedges or slices. Separate lettuce leaves; arrange them on a large serving platter. Top with eggs, celery, tomatoes, and chicken. Drizzle with dressing. Refrigerate remaining dressing for another use.

PER SERVING: 200 calories, 14 g fat (4 g saturated fat), 16 g protein, 880 mg sodium, 8 g carbohydrates, 6 g sugars (0 g added sugars), 2 g fiber

Tip **Looking to up your ratios? Add an ounce of crumbled blue cheese to each serving.**

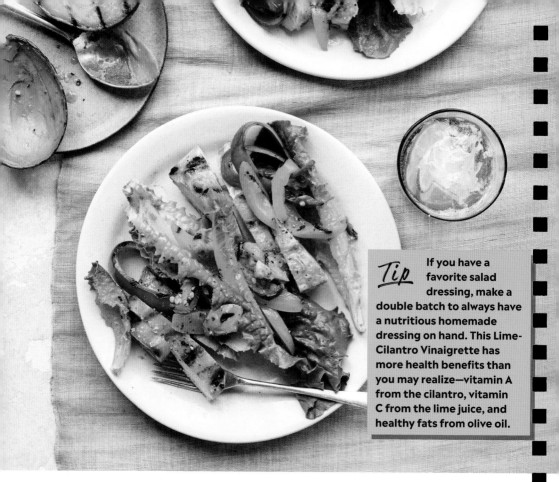

Chicken Fajita Salad with Lime-Cilantro Vinaigrette

Active time: 35 minutes
Total time: 35 minutes
Makes: 4 servings

→ This veggie-packed take on chicken fajitas makes a typically high-caloric dish keto-approved. Plus, chicken breasts are an excellent source of protein—one portion contains almost half of your daily requirement.

INGREDIENTS

- ✪ 2 8-ounce boneless, skinless chicken breasts
- Kosher salt and black pepper
- 2 bell peppers (orange and yellow), quartered lengthwise
- 1 jalapeño, halved lengthwise
- ✪ 1 medium onion, sliced into ½-inch-thick rounds
- 3 tablespoon plus 1 teaspoon olive oil
- ✪ 1 avocado
- ✪ 2 limes
- 2 packed cups cilantro (including thin stems)
- 2 small hearts romaine, leaves separated, halved if large

1. Heat a grill to medium-high. Season chicken with ¼ teaspoon each salt and black pepper.

2. In a large bowl, toss bell peppers, jalapeño, and onion with 1 tablespoon olive oil and season with ¼ teaspoon each salt and black pepper. Cut avocado in half, remove pit, and gently rub flesh with 1 teaspoon olive oil.

3. Grill chicken until cooked through, 7 to 8 minutes per side; transfer to a cutting board. Grill vegetables until just tender, 4 to 6 minutes per side, transferring to a cutting board as they are done. Grill avocado, cut sides down, until charred, 1 to 2 minutes.

4. Slice peppers and jalapeño, separate onions into rings, and dice avocado.

5. Finely grate zest of 1 lime into a blender. Squeeze in 6 tablespoons lime juice. Add cilantro and 2 tablespoons olive oil and puree dressing until smooth.

6. Toss romaine with ¼ cup dressing. Slice chicken; divide among plates along with peppers, jalapeño, onion, and avocado. Serve with remaining dressing.

PER SERVING: 360 calories, 21.5 g fat (3.5 g saturated fat), 26 g protein, 315 mg sodium, 17 g carbohydrates, 5 g sugars (0 g added sugars), 6 g fiber

Ratatouille Salad

Active time: 20 minutes
Total time: 20 minutes
Makes: 4 servings

→ Ratatouille could be considered the winning recipe of nutritious vegetables. Bell peppers and eggplant are just two of the healthy veggies always highlighted in this dish. Red bell peppers contain more than 200 percent of your Recommended Daily Intake of vitamin C, while eggplants are high in fiber, which helps control your blood sugar.

INGREDIENTS

1 red bell pepper, quartered
1 small eggplant (about 12 ounces), sliced into ¼-inch-thick rounds
1 medium zucchini (about 6 ounces), sliced lengthwise into ¼-inch-thick planks
1 small summer squash (about 6 ounces), sliced lengthwise into ¼-inch-thick planks
✪ 1 pound Campari or plum tomatoes, halved
✪ 2 ½ tablespoons olive oil
Kosher salt and pepper
2 tablespoons red wine vinegar
¼ cup basil leaves, torn
✪ 4 cups baby arugula
✪ 1 clove garlic, halved
2 ounces fresh mozzarella, torn

1. Heat a grill to medium-high.

2. In a large bowl, toss vegetables with 1½ tablespoons olive oil and ½ teaspoon each salt and pepper. Grill until lightly charred and tender, 3 to 4 minutes per side for bell pepper, eggplant, zucchini, and squash and 1 to 2 minutes on cut sides only for tomatoes. Return eggplant and tomatoes to bowl and transfer rest of vegetables to a cutting board.

3. Slice bell pepper, zucchini, and squash and add to bowl. Gently toss with vinegar, basil, and arugula. Divide salad between 4 plates and top each plate with mozzarella before serving.

PER SERVING: 192 calories, 13 g fat (3 g saturated fat), 7 g protein, 273 mg sodium, 16 g carbohydrates, 10 g sugars (0 g added sugars), 6 g fiber

Spiced Grilled Eggplant & Tomatoes

Active time: 15 minutes
Total time: 30 minutes
Makes: 6 servings

→ If you don't like the texture of eggplant you've eaten, prepare it another way. Grilling eggplant brings out the vegetable's natural sugars, making it less bitter and allowing it to stay firm. Eggplants are rich in anthocyanins, which are responsible for its skin's bright pigment and also act as an antioxidant that can protect cells from free radicals, reducing the risk of diseases such as cancer and cardiovascular disease.

INGREDIENTS

- 2 medium eggplants (about 1 pound each), sliced lengthwise ½ inch thick
- ✪ 4 tablespoons olive oil
- 1 teaspoon ground coriander
- 1 teaspoon cayenne
- Kosher salt
- ✪ 2 tablespoons fresh lemon juice
- 2 tablespoons red wine vinegar
- ✪ 1½ cups cherry or grape tomatoes in different colors, halved
- 2 small Fresno chiles or other hot chiles, finely chopped
- ¼ cup packed mint leaves, finely chopped, plus more for topping
- ✪ ¼ cup low-fat Greek yogurt
- 2 tablespoons low-fat milk

1. Heat a grill to medium. Brush eggplant with 3 tablespoons olive oil, then season with coriander, cayenne, and ¼ teaspoon salt. Grill until tender, 10 to 12 minutes.

2. Meanwhile, in a medium bowl, whisk together lemon juice, vinegar, 1 tablespoon olive oil, and ¼ teaspoon salt; fold in tomatoes, chiles, and mint.

3. Arrange eggplant on a large platter; top with tomato salad. Whisk together yogurt and milk and drizzle over vegetables. Sprinkle with mint, if desired.

PER SERVING: 141 calories, 10 g fat (1.5 g saturated fat), 3 g protein, 308 mg sodium, 12 g carbohydrates, 6g sugars (0g added sugars), 5g fiber

---

Tip
Zucchini is a popular low-carb substitution but eggplant is a low-carb alternative that tends to receive less attention. Use eggplant in place of lasagna noodles or even as the "bread" for an open-faced sandwich. The rich, meaty flavor will be just as satisfying.

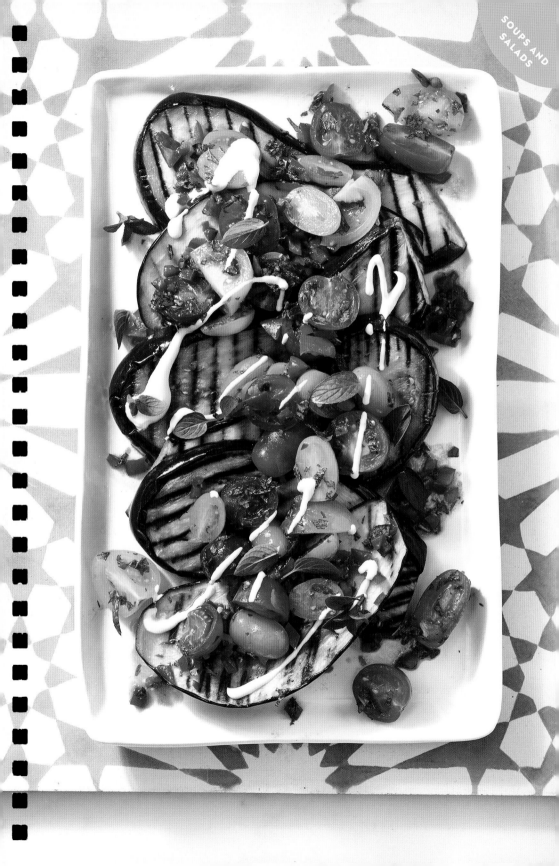

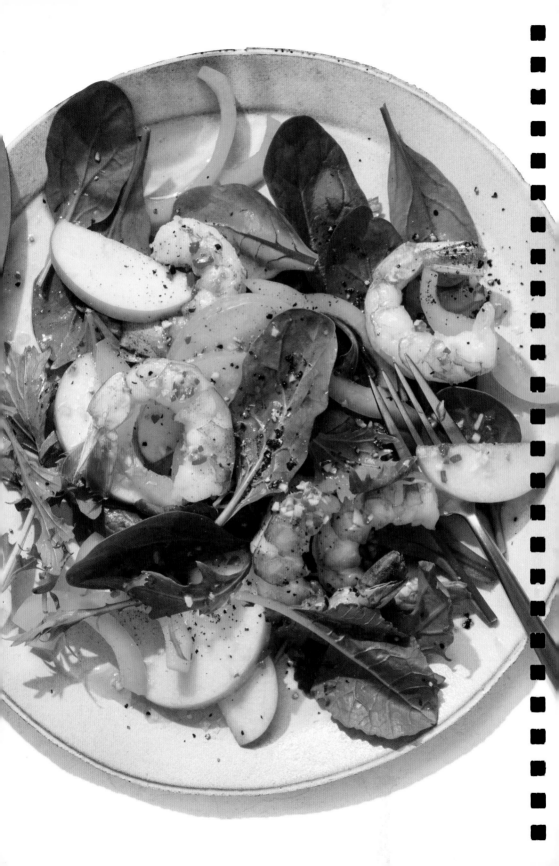

Shrimp Salad with Chile Vinaigrette

Active time: 15 minutes
Total time: 15 minutes
Makes: 4 servings

→ Shrimp is a low-carb power protein that has properties to aid in weight loss as well as anti-aging. Who knew? The high levels of zinc in shrimp help to produce the hormone called leptin, which helps control energy use in the body. Astaxanthin is an antioxidant in shrimp that has been found to reduce aging from UVA damage.

INGREDIENTS

- ✪ 1 lemon
- 2 cups water
- ✪ ½ pound peeled and deveined shrimp
- ✪ 3 tablespoons extra-virgin olive oil
- 1 tablespoon white wine vinegar
- ½ teaspoon kosher salt
- 1 Fresno chile, finely chopped
- 1 clove garlic, finely chopped
- 1 Granny Smith apple, thinly sliced
- 1 yellow bell pepper, thinly sliced
- ✪ 1 5-ounce package power greens such as spinach, baby kale, chard, or collards

1. Halve lemon, squeeze, and set aside 1 tablespoon juice. Place halves in a large pot, add 2 cups water, and bring to a simmer. Place a steamer basket in the pot, add shrimp, cover, and steam until shrimp are opaque throughout, about 4 minutes; transfer to a bowl of ice water to cool. Drain shrimp and pat dry.

2. In a large bowl, whisk together olive oil, vinegar, reserved lemon juice, and salt; stir in Fresno chile and garlic.

3. Add apple and yellow pepper slices and cooled shrimp. Toss to coat, then fold in power greens.

PER SERVING: 200 calories, 11.5 g fat (1.5 g saturated fat), 11 g protein, 650 mg sodium, 14 g carbohydrates, 7.5 g sugars (3 g added sugars), 2 g fiber

Tip When buying shrimp, look for varieties that are already peeled and deveined for easy preparation. If the shrimp is not deveined, this process is simple. Use a paring knife to make a long slit along the back of the shrimp and simply pull the vein out. You are actually removing the shrimp's digestive tract!

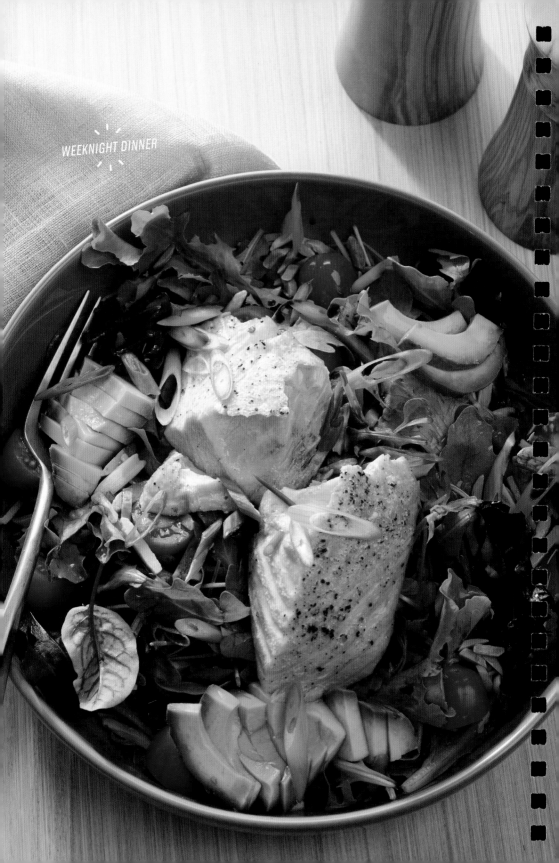

Wild Salmon Salad

Active time: 15 minutes
Total time: 15 minutes
Makes: 4 servings

→ There's much to love about this power salad. The healthy omega-3s from the salmon and unsaturated fat from the avocado are two of the best types of fat to keep your stomach full and your mind happy.

INGREDIENTS

- ✪ 4 4-ounce pieces skinless wild Alaskan salmon fillet
- Kosher salt and pepper
- 2 tablespoons balsamic vinegar
- 2 teaspoons olive oil
- ✪ 1 pint grape tomatoes, halved
- ✪ 2 scallions, thinly sliced
- ✪ ½ cup slivered almonds, toasted
- 5 ounces mixed baby greens
- ✪ 1 avocado, sliced

1. Heat oven to 375°F. Season salmon with ½ teaspoon each salt and pepper, place on a rimmed baking sheet, and roast until opaque throughout, 10 to 12 minutes.

2. Meanwhile, in a large bowl, whisk together vinegar, olive oil, and a pinch each salt and pepper. Toss with tomatoes; fold in scallions and almonds. Toss with greens and avocado. Serve with salmon.

PER SERVING: 340 calories, 20.5 g fat (3 g saturated fat), 28 g protein, 350 mg sodium, 13 g carbohydrates, 4.5 g sugars (0 g added sugars), 7 g fiber

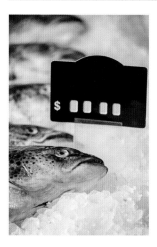

WILD VS. FARM-RAISED SALMON

When shopping for salmon, it's important to look for the wild variety rather than farm-raised. Farm-raised salmon eats a processed fish feed during its lifetime rather than organisms found in its natural habitat. As a result, wild salmon is higher in minerals such as potassium and iron, and tends to be lower in calories than farm-raised salmon. Farm-raised salmon often has fewer nutrients, higher levels of disease-causing pesticides, and higher amounts of saturated fat than wild salmon. And when it comes to taste there is no comparison: Wild salmon has a richer flavor, making it a clear winner.

Roasted Cauliflower "Steak" Salad

Active time: 10 minutes
Total time: 60 minutes
Makes: 4 servings

→ Raw dandelion greens contain antioxidants that may help reduce inflammation. Look for younger, smaller greens found in the spring. If only bunches of larger dandelion greens are available (and you don't like the extra-bitter bite), opt for arugula instead.

INGREDIENTS

- 2 tablespoons olive oil
- 2 large heads cauliflower (about 3 pounds each), trimmed of outer leaves
- 2 teaspoons za'atar
- 1 ½ teaspoons kosher salt
- 1 ¼ teaspoons black pepper
- 1 teaspoon ground cumin
- 2 large carrots
- 8 ounces dandelion greens, tough stems removed
- ✪ ½ cup plain low-fat Greek yogurt
- 2 tablespoons tahini
- ✪ 2 tablespoons fresh lemon juice
- ✪ 1 clove garlic, minced

1. Heat oven to 450°F. Brush a large baking sheet with some of the olive oil.

2. Place 1 cauliflower head on a cutting board, stem side down. Cut down the middle, through core and stem, and then cut 2 1-inch-thick "steaks" from middle. Repeat with the other cauliflower head. Set aside remaining cauliflower for another use. Brush both sides of steaks with remaining olive oil and set on baking sheet.

3. Combine za'atar, 1 teaspoon salt, 1 teaspoon pepper, and cumin. Sprinkle on cauliflower steaks. Bake until bottom is deeply golden, about 30 minutes. Flip and bake until tender, 10 to 15 minutes.

4. Meanwhile, set carrots on the cutting board and use a vegetable peeler to peel into ribbons. Place in a large bowl with dandelion greens.

5. In small bowl, combine yogurt, tahini, lemon juice, 1 tablespoon water, ½ teaspoon salt, ¼ teaspoon pepper, and garlic.

6. Dab 3 tablespoons of dressing onto carrot-dandelion mix. With a spoon or your hands, massage dressing into mix, about 5 minutes.

7. Remove steaks from oven and transfer to individual plates. Drizzle each with 2 tablespoons of dressing and top with 1 cup of salad.

PER SERVING: 214 calories, 12 g fat (2 g saturated fat), 9 g protein, 849 mg sodium, 21 g carbohydrates, 8 g sugars (0 g added sugars), 7 g fiber

Tip Tahini is a very nutritious ingredient that looks similar to peanut butter. It is made from ground sesame seeds and has a rich, nutty flavor. Tahini is a good source of protein and heart-healthy fats and also contains B vitamins that help with energy function. Be careful, though, as tahini is fairly high in calories—but good news: Just a little bit of this nutty spread goes a long way in terms of flavor.

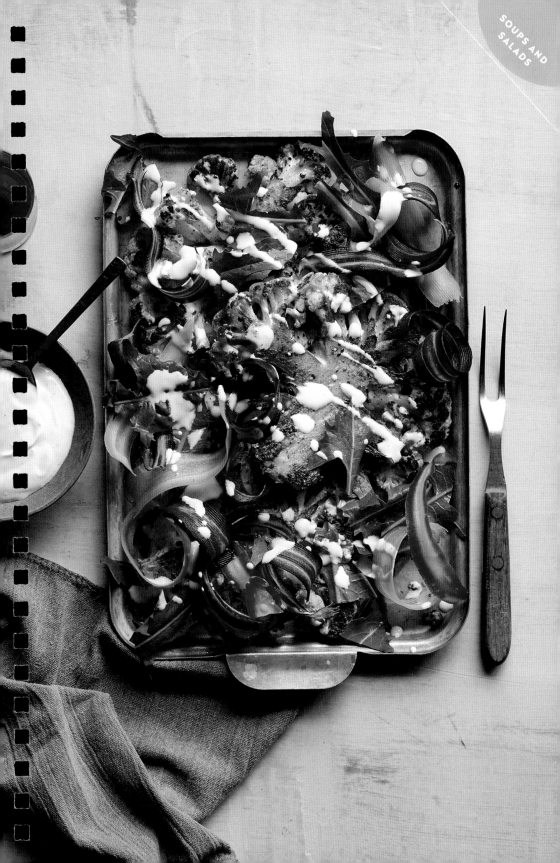

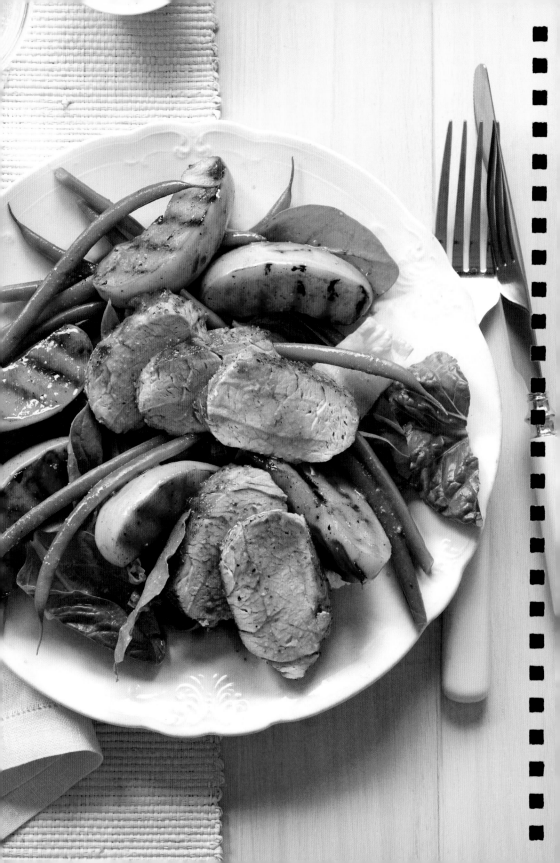

Grilled Pork & Apple Salad

Active time: 15 minutes
Total time: 35 minutes
Makes: 4 servings

→ Green beans are a veggie side-dish staple. Grilling the green beans adds a smoky twist to the standard steamed option. Plus, green beans are full of fiber, to help with gastrointestinal issues, and folic acid, which is essential for pregnant women and can also help increase fertility.

INGREDIENTS

8 ounces green beans
2 Gala apples, sliced
3 teaspoons sugar-free
   maple syrup
✪ 1 tablespoon plus
   2 teaspoons olive oil
1 whole pork tenderloin
Salt and pepper
1 romaine lettuce heart
2 tablespoons balsamic
   vinegar
1 teaspoon Dijon mustard
✪ 6 ounces baby spinach

1. Prepare a grill for covered direct grilling on medium.

2. Place beans on a 16-by-12-inch sheet of heavy-duty foil. Fold in half; crimp foil edges to create a sealed packet. Toss apples with 1 teaspoon each maple syrup and olive oil. Rub 1 teaspoon olive oil all over pork, then sprinkle with ¼ teaspoon each salt and black pepper.

3. Place packet, apples, and pork on grill; cover. Grill apples for 8 minutes, turning once. Transfer apples to a large bowl; let cool. Grill beans for 10 minutes. Transfer packet to a plate; open and let cool. Grill pork, turning occasionally, until an instant-read thermometer inserted into pork registers 145°F, about 15 minutes. Transfer to a cutting board; let rest 10 minutes.

4. Chop lettuce. In a large bowl, whisk vinegar, mustard, 1 tablespoon olive oil, 2 teaspoons maple syrup, and ⅛ teaspoon each salt and pepper. Add spinach, lettuce, green beans, and apples; toss well. Thinly slice pork across the grain. Serve with salad.

PER SERVING: 135 calories, 6 g fat (1 g saturated fat), 5 g protein, 100 mg sodium, 15 g carbohydrates, 3 g fiber, 10 g sugars (0 g added sugar)

Bacon & Egg Salad

Active time: 10 minutes
Total time: 40 minutes
Makes: 4 servings

→ This salad could be for brunch, lunch, or dinner and is genius because it uses the bacon fat as the base for the salad dressing. And you know what that means: The salad will not only keep you in ketosis but will have that delicious smoky bacon flavor in every bite.

INGREDIENTS

4 slices bacon, diced
1 large shallot, minced
¼ cup sherry vinegar
✪ 2 tablespoons olive oil
2 tablespoons chopped parsley
1 tablespoon chopped thyme leaves
2 teaspoons Dijon mustard
½ teaspoon kosher salt
½ teaspoon black pepper
½ pound asparagus, trimmed
✪ 4 large eggs
✪ 6 cups baby arugula
2 tablespoons grated Parmesan, for topping

1. Cook bacon in a skillet until crisp, about 8 minutes. Transfer to a plate. Remove all but 2 tablespoons bacon fat from skillet, reduce heat, and add shallot. Cook until tender, about 4 minutes. Add vinegar, scraping up crispy bits. Remove from heat and stir in olive oil, parsley, thyme, mustard, salt, and pepper.

2. Fill a large saucepan halfway with water and bring to a low simmer. Add asparagus and cook until crisp-tender, about 2 minutes. Remove asparagus and set aside. Return water to a simmer, then crack in 1 egg. Cook until white is set but yolk is runny, about 4 minutes. Remove with a slotted spoon. Repeat with remaining eggs.

3. Toss arugula with dressing. Divide among 4 plates and top with asparagus, eggs, bacon, and cheese.

PER SERVING: 277 calories, 22 g fat (6.5 g saturated fat), 13 g protein, 568 mg sodium, 7 g carbohydrates, 3 g sugars (0 g added sugars), 2 g fiber

Tip **When shopping for asparagus** it's best to go for the skinnier stalks. If all you can find is thick asparagus, be sure to discard the woody bottoms and remove the outer layer of the asparagus using a vegetable peeler. This will help your tough asparagus become more tender as it cooks.

BRUNCH
PICK

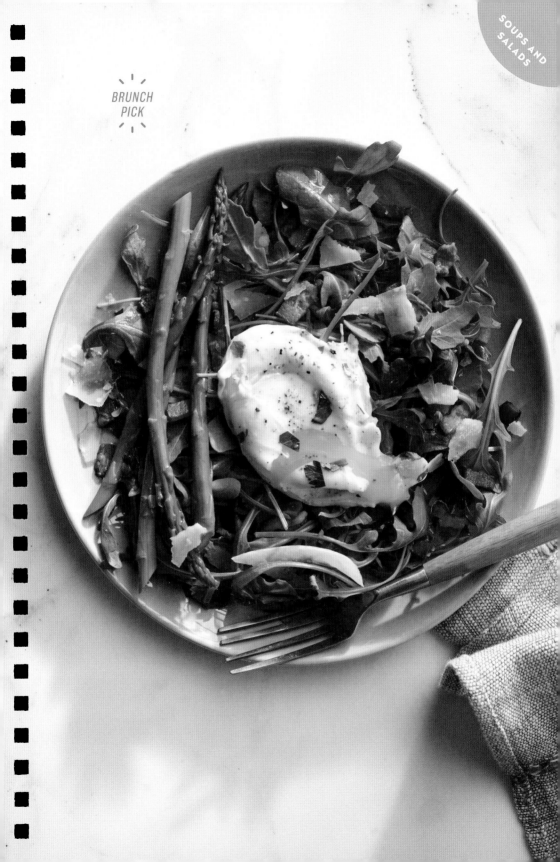

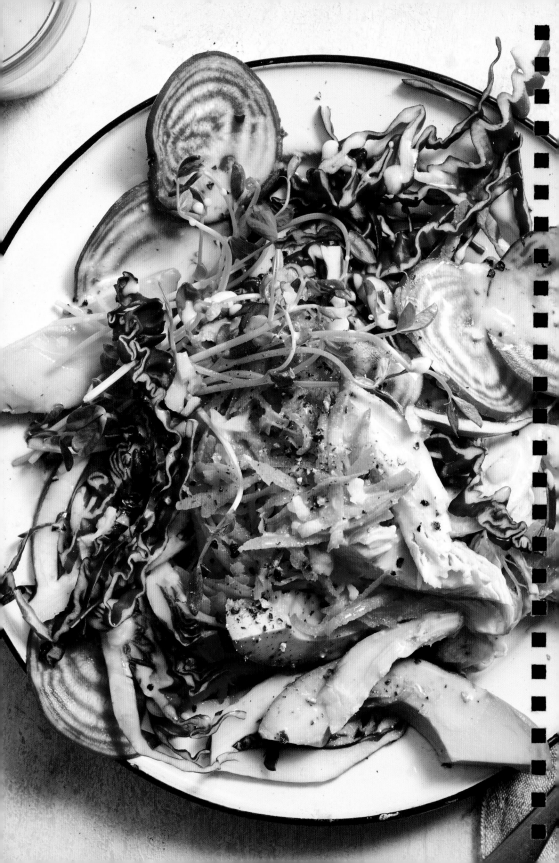

Rainbow Chicken Slaw

Active time: 20 minutes
Total time: 20 minutes
Makes: 2 servings

→ Beta-carotene is an antioxidant found in both carrots and snow pea shoots. Beta-carotene is converted into vitamin A, which supports the immune system, eye health, and skin. It also helps protect the body from free radicals, which destroy your cells and cause illness.

INGREDIENTS

½ cup low-fat buttermilk
4 teaspoons fresh lemon juice
2 small cloves garlic, finely grated
2 teaspoons honey mustard
Kosher salt and pepper
✪ 1½ cups shredded cooked chicken
1 cup thinly sliced red cabbage
2 small carrots, coarsely grated
2 small rainbow or Chioggia beets, scrubbed and very thinly sliced
✪ 1 avocado, sliced
½ cup snow pea shoots

1. In a medium bowl, whisk together buttermilk, lemon juice, garlic, honey mustard, and ¼ teaspoon pepper. Transfer half of dressing to a small bowl and set aside. Add chicken to remaining bowl of dressing and toss to coat.

2. Arrange cabbage, carrots, beets, avocado, and pea shoots on 2 large plates and season to taste with salt and pepper. Top with chicken and drizzle with remaining dressing, tossing before eating.

PER SERVING: 460 calories, 24.5 g fat (4.5 g saturated fat), 32 g protein, 740 mg sodium, 33 g carbohydrates, 16.5 g sugars (1.5 g added sugars), 12 g fiber

Tip It is important not to consume too much vitamin A, because extremely high levels can actually become toxic to the body.

91

Chapter 4

Mains

And now for the star of the dinnertime show—the entrée. When planning your evening meals on the keto diet, it's important to have enough fat and protein to keep you satisfied until the next meal in the morning. Sometimes diet recipes can be hard or even boring at dinnertime, especially when others at the table would rather eat something else. Luckily, these simple recipes are packed with flavor and nutrients to keep everyone happy—and there's a recipe to fit anyone's craving. For a delicious Asian option, try the Chicken Fried "Rice," or if you are feeling Italian, the "Spaghetti" and Meatballs. Need a fancier course for entertaining? Try the Parchment-Baked Halibut with Fennel and Carrots or the Glazed Bacon-Wrapped Turkey Breast to keep you on track and your guests impressed.

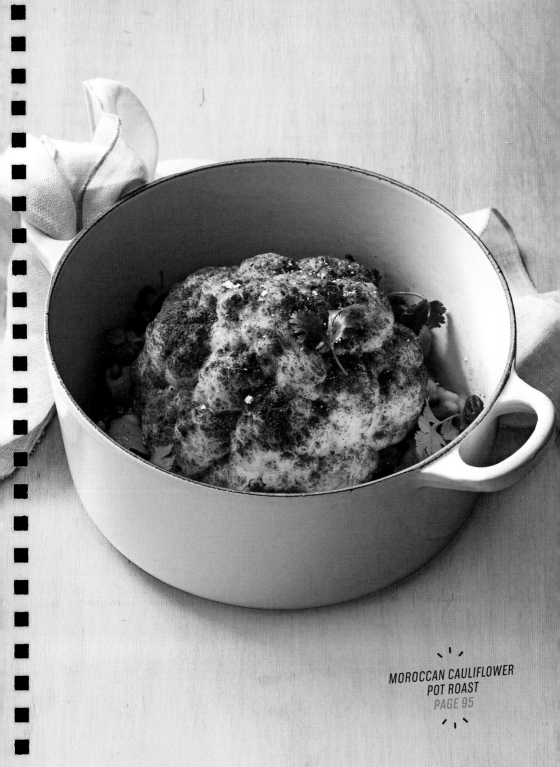

MOROCCAN CAULIFLOWER
POT ROAST
PAGE 95

Eggplant & Parmesan "Meatballs"

Active time: 35 minutes
Total time: 1 hour
Makes: 5 servings

- ✪ 1 tablespoon olive oil
- ✪ 2 cloves garlic, finely chopped
- 1¼ pounds eggplant, cut into 1-inch pieces
- Kosher salt and pepper
- Cooking spray, for the pan
- 1¾ cups almond flour
- 2 oz Parmesan, finely grated (½ to ¾ cup)
- ½ cup flat-leaf parsley, finely chopped
- ¼ cup basil leaves, finely chopped
- ✪ 1 large egg, beaten
- 2 cups low-sodium marinara sauce

1. Heat oil and garlic in a large skillet on medium until it sizzles, 3 minutes. Add eggplant, ¼ cup water, and ¼ teaspoon each salt and pepper and cook, covered, on medium-low, stirring occasionally, until tender, 12 to 15 minutes. Transfer to a colander and let drain 5 minutes.

2. Meanwhile, heat oven to 400°F; line a baking sheet with nonstick foil; lightly coat with nonstick cooking spray.

3. Transfer eggplant mixture to a food processor and pulse to roughly chop (do not puree). Add almond flour, Parmesan, parsley, basil, and ½ teaspoon each salt and pepper; pulse to combine.

4. Stir in egg. Form into twenty 1½-inch balls and transfer to prepared baking sheet. Bake until firm and browned on the bottom, 15 to 20 minutes.

5. Heat sauce in a large skillet, then gently toss in meatballs.

PER SERVING 396 calories, 29.5 g fat (4 g saturated fat), 15 g protein, 687 mg sodium, 23 g carbohydrates, 8 g sugars (0 g added sugars), 10 g fiber

 Tip Missing the noodles? Serve these veggie-forward "meatballs" over spaghetti squash or zoodles for a low-carb alternative.

Moroccan Cauliflower Pot Roast

Active time: 10 minutes
Total time: 1 hour 15 minutes
Makes: 4 servings

→ You won't even notice there's no meat in this pot roast. The blend of rich and health-benefiting spices gives the fiber-loaded cauliflower a decadent flavor for a plant-based dish that will keep you feeling full and satisfied.

INGREDIENTS
2 teaspoons ground coriander
1½ teaspoons ground cumin
1½ teaspoons chile powder
1 teaspoon turmeric
½ teaspoon ground cinnamon
½ teaspoon kosher salt
½ teaspoon black pepper
1 large head cauliflower
✪ 3 teaspoons olive oil
✪ 1 onion, sliced into ½-inch wedges
1 clove garlic, sliced
2 cups reduced-sodium vegetable broth

1. Heat oven to 375°F. In a small bowl, combine coriander, cumin, chile powder, turmeric, cinnamon, salt, and pepper.

2. Slice stalk from cauliflower so it sits flat; score bottom with an X. Brush with 1½ teaspoons olive oil; coat with spice rub. Heat 1½ teaspoons olive oil in a large heavy pot on medium. Add onion and garlic. Cook until onion begins to soften, 5 minutes. Add broth, bring to a simmer, and place cauliflower in pot, spice side up.

3. Cover pot and bake 30 minutes. Remove cover; bake until cauliflower is tender, 25 to 30 minutes more. Slice cauliflower into wedges and serve with onion mix and liquid.

PER SERVING: 114 calories, 4.5 g fat (1 g saturated fat), 5 g protein, 405 mg sodium, 17 g carbohydrates, 6 g sugars (0 g added sugars), 6 g fiber

Spaghetti Squash Bowls

Active time: 10 minutes
Total time: 1 hour 20 minutes
Makes: 4 servings

→ A great noodle alternative, spaghetti squash becomes slightly sweet when roasted and makes a perfect base for sauces, cheese, and herbs. Plus, it's low-calorie and high in fiber and vitamin C, helping you keep your digestion on track. After enjoying this dish you might even ask, "Who needs spaghetti?"

INGREDIENTS

2 small spaghetti squash (about 3 pounds each), halved and seeded
16 ounces part-skim ricotta
✪ 10 ounces frozen chopped spinach, thawed and squeezed dry
¼ cup sliced pitted kalamata olives
2 tablespoons chopped oregano leaves
✪ 4 teaspoons lemon zest
✪ 4 teaspoons olive oil
½ teaspoon kosher salt
½ teaspoon black pepper
✪ 4 teaspoons pine nuts, toasted, for topping
1 ounce Pecorino, shaved, for topping

1. Heat oven to 425°F. Place squash halves, cut side down, in a baking dish. Add 2 cups water and cover tightly with foil. Bake until squash is tender, 30 minutes. Leave oven on.

2. Let squash cool slightly. Using a fork, scrape flesh into a large bowl; reserve shell halves. Stir in ricotta, spinach, olives, oregano, lemon zest, olive oil, salt, and pepper.

3. Divide mixture among 4 squash halves and bake until bubbly, 20 minutes more. Top with pine nuts and Pecorino.

PER SERVING: 387 calories, 25 g fat (8 g saturated fat), 20 g protein, 916 mg sodium, 24 g carbohydrates, 5 g sugars (0 g added sugars), 5 g fiber

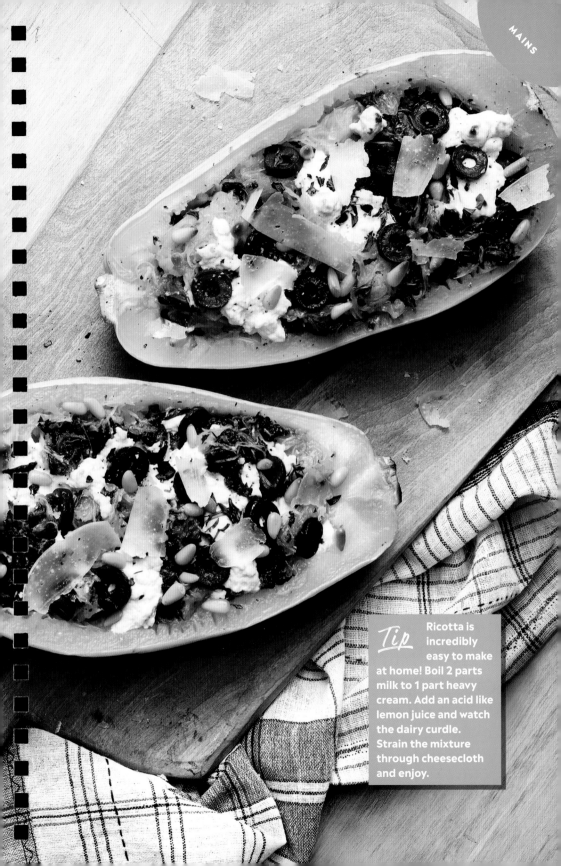

Tip Ricotta is incredibly easy to make at home! Boil 2 parts milk to 1 part heavy cream. Add an acid like lemon juice and watch the dairy curdle. Strain the mixture through cheesecloth and enjoy.

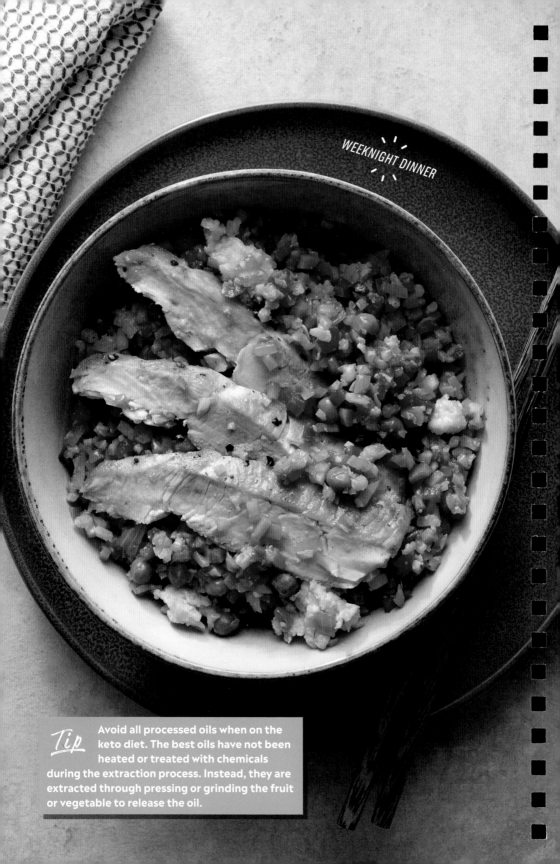

WEEKNIGHT DINNER

Tip Avoid all processed oils when on the keto diet. The best oils have not been heated or treated with chemicals during the extraction process. Instead, they are extracted through pressing or grinding the fruit or vegetable to release the oil.

Chicken Fried "Rice"

Active time: 25 minutes
Total time: 25 minutes
Makes: 4 servings

→ If you love the fried rice from your local Chinese restaurant, try this recipe. It's packed with all the same delicious veggies and salty flavor, but without the heavy carbs.

INGREDIENTS

- ✪ 1 tablespoon plus 2 teaspoons avocado oil
- ✪ ½ pound boneless, skinless chicken breast, pounded to even thickness
- ✪ 2 large eggs, beaten
- 1 red bell pepper, finely chopped
- 1 small carrot, finely chopped
- ✪ ½ small onion, finely chopped
- ✪ 1 clove garlic, finely chopped
- 2 scallions, finely chopped, plus more for serving
- ½ cup frozen peas, thawed
- 2 cups cauliflower "rice"
- 1 tablespoon coconut aminos
- 1 teaspoon rice vinegar
- Kosher salt and pepper

1. Heat a large, deep skillet on medium-high. When hot, add 1 tablespoon avocado oil, then chicken, and cook until chicken is golden brown, 3 to 4 minutes per side. Transfer to a cutting board and let rest 6 minutes before slicing.

2. Add 2 teaspoons avocado oil to skillet, then eggs, and scramble, about 1 minute; transfer to a bowl.

3. Add red pepper, carrot, and onion to skillet and cook, stirring often, until just tender, 4 to 5 minutes. Stir in garlic and cook 1 minute. Add scallions and peas to the skillet and toss to combine.

4. Add cauliflower, coconut aminos, and rice vinegar and toss to combine. Let cauliflower sit, without stirring, 2 minutes. Toss with chicken, eggs, and ¼ teaspoon each salt and pepper.

PER SERVING: 210 calories, 10 g fat (2 g saturated fat), 19 g protein, 340 mg sodium, 10 g carbohydrates, 5 g sugars (0 g added sugars), 4 g fiber

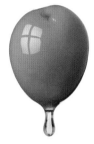

COOKING OILS FOR KETO

Olive oil is a great keto cooking oil to have on hand. It's rich in heart-healthy monounsaturated fats that lower "bad" LDL cholesterol and raise "good" HDL cholesterol. But you can also experiment with other cooking oils such as sesame oil, avocado oil, and coconut oil. Sesame oil has a rich and nutty flavor that's great for Asian dishes, and it contains vitamins E and B6. Avocado oil is high in monounsaturated acids, just like olive oil, and boasts anti-inflammatory properties, like the fruit does. Both sesame and avocado oils have a high smoke point for cooking. Coconut oil has shorter fatty acid chains that are used by the body more quickly. This helps to increase metabolism and keep you in ketosis. Coconut oil tends to have a lower smoke point than the other oils, so it should be used in low and slow cooking methods.

Chicken Caprese

Active time: 15 minutes
Total time: 25 minutes
Makes: 4 servings

→ Mozarella provides gooey goodness in this classic Italian recipe and ups your ratios, too.

INGREDIENTS
- 3 tablespoons olive oil
- 4 chicken breast cutlets (about 1 ¼ pounds)
- 1 ¼ pounds tomatoes, chopped
- 3 cloves garlic, sliced
- ½ teaspoon kosher salt
- 8 ounces mini fresh mozzarella balls, halved
- 2 tablespoons chopped basil leaves
- Roasted or steamed Broccolini, for serving

1. Heat olive oil in a 12-inch skillet on medium-high; add chicken and cook, turning once, until cooked through (165°F), about 6 minutes. Transfer cutlets to a plate and cover to keep warm.

2. To the skillet, add tomatoes, garlic, and salt. Cook 3 minutes, stirring and scraping.

3. Top chicken with tomato sauce, mozzarella balls, and basil leaves. Serve with roasted or steamed Broccolini.

PER SERVING: 475 calories, 28 g fat (10 g saturated fat), 45 g protein, 570 mg sodium, 12 g carbohydrates, 0 g sugars (0 g added sugars), 4 g fiber

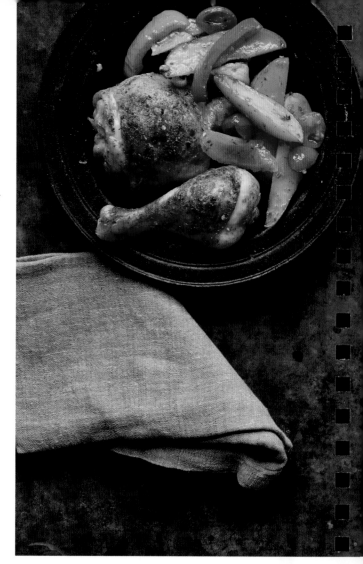

Pollo Alla Calabrese

Active time: 10 minutes
Total time: 1 hour
Makes: 4 servings

→ This convenient one-pan meal from the Calabrian region of southern Italy is full of nutrients and protein. Bell peppers contain an abundance of water, which aids hydration, but also have the added benefits of vitamin B6, which helps form red blood cells, and vitamin K1, good for bone health and blood clotting.

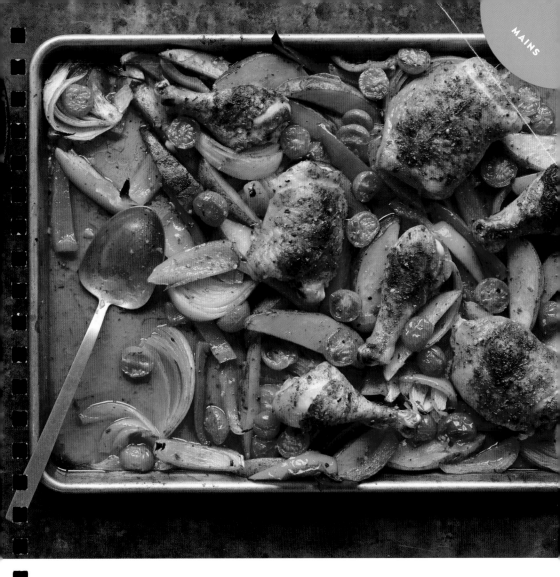

INGREDIENTS

- 4 chicken drumsticks
- 4 bone-in, skin-on chicken thighs
- ❂ 1 pint cherry tomatoes, halved
- 3 red, orange, or yellow bell peppers, cut into ½-inch strips
- ❂ 1 large sweet onion, cut into ½-inch wedges
- ❂ ¼ cup olive oil
- ❂ 4 cloves garlic, minced
- 1 teaspoon dried oregano
- 1 teaspoon sweet paprika
- 1 teaspoon kosher salt
- ¼ teaspoon red pepper flakes

1. Heat oven to 400°F.

2. On a large rimmed baking sheet, combine chicken, tomatoes, bell peppers, onion, olive oil, garlic, oregano, paprika, salt, and red pepper flakes, tossing to combine and rubbing chicken with spices.

3. Arrange vegetables underneath chicken pieces. Roast, turning chicken and tossing vegetables halfway through, until vegetables are tender and a thermometer inserted in thickest part of chicken, but not touching bone, registers 165°F, about 45 minutes.

PER SERVING: 571 calories, 23 g fat (6 g saturated fat), 56 g protein, 755 mg sodium, 34 g carbohydrates, 11 g sugars (0 g added sugars), 6 g fiber

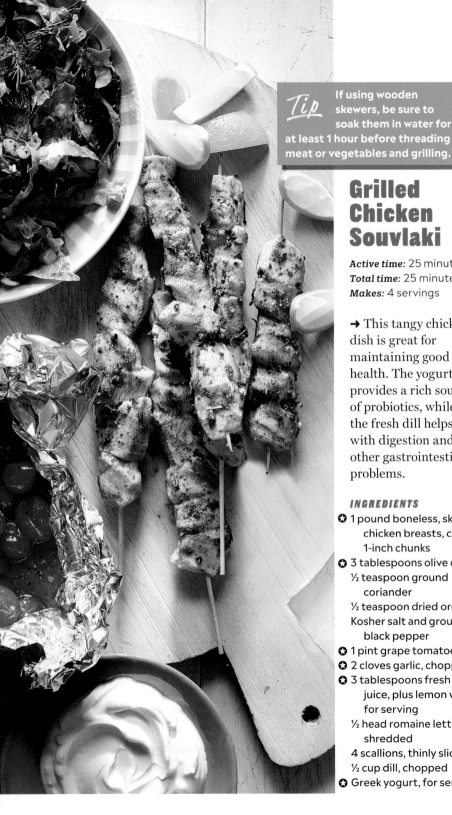

Tip If using wooden skewers, be sure to soak them in water for at least 1 hour before threading meat or vegetables and grilling.

Grilled Chicken Souvlaki

Active time: 25 minutes
Total time: 25 minutes
Makes: 4 servings

→ This tangy chicken dish is great for maintaining good gut health. The yogurt provides a rich source of probiotics, while the fresh dill helps with digestion and other gastrointestinal problems.

INGREDIENTS

- ✪ 1 pound boneless, skinless chicken breasts, cut into 1-inch chunks
- ✪ 3 tablespoons olive oil
- ½ teaspoon ground coriander
- ½ teaspoon dried oregano
- Kosher salt and ground black pepper
- ✪ 1 pint grape tomatoes
- ✪ 2 cloves garlic, chopped
- ✪ 3 tablespoons fresh lemon juice, plus lemon wedges for serving
- ½ head romaine lettuce, shredded
- 4 scallions, thinly sliced
- ½ cup dill, chopped
- ✪ Greek yogurt, for serving

1. Preheat a grill on medium-high. In a medum bowl, toss chicken with 1 tablespoon olive oil, then add coriander, oregano, and ¼ teaspoon each salt and pepper; toss. Thread chicken onto skewers.

2. Place tomatoes and garlic on a large piece of heavy-duty foil. Sprinkle with 1 tablespoon olive oil and ¼ teaspoon each salt and pepper. Fold and crimp the foil to form a pouch.

3. Place pouch and skewers on the grill. Cook, shaking the pouch and turning the skewers occasionally, until chicken is cooked through, 8 to 10 minutes. Just before removing it from the grill, brush chicken with 1 tablespoon of lemon juice.

4. Meanwhile, in a bowl, toss lettuce, scallions, and dill with 2 tablespoons lemon juice, 1 tablespoon olive oil, and ¼ teaspoon each salt and pepper.

5. Serve chicken topped with Greek yogurt and tomatoes, along with salad and lemon wedges.

PER SERVING:
About 245 calories, 13 g fat
(2 g saturated fat), 25 g protein,
426 mg sodium,
8 g carbohydrates, 4 g sugars
(0 g added sugars), 3 g fiber

HEALTHY FLAVOR HACKS

Unfortunately, diet food is usually considered bland and boring. But this should never be a problem. Add these simple fresh ingredients that are low in carbs but big on flavor.

HOT CHILE PEPPERS
Fresh or dry, the spiciness in hot peppers works in two ways. It adds flavor to dishes like stir-fries, but it also slows you down. Making mealtime a mindful experience can help you eat less overall.

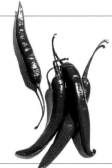

GRAPEFRUIT
Citrus's acidity helps you cut back on salt and sugar. Pair grapefruit with meat, seafood, or salad—you'll add antioxidants and fiber and say goodbye to unhealthier store-bought dressings and marinades.

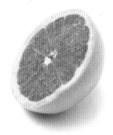

CHIVES
Onion's little cousins add plenty of bold aromatic flavor. That's good for your taste buds and also helps you rein in the salt.

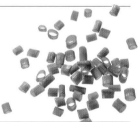

TOMATO PASTE
This adds tangy, hearty flavor to sautés, sauces, and soups. Slash your sodium intake by choosing brands that say "no salt added," then sprinkle in a little salt of your own.

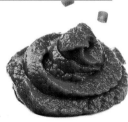

Portobello Turkey Burger with Bruschetta Topping

Active time: 10 minutes
Total time: 20 minutes
Makes: 1 serving

→ You could call this burger magic, because that's what it is! Portobello mushrooms work as the perfect low-carb substitute for a regular hamburger bun. Better yet, mushrooms have awesome health benefits, like lowering cholesterol, and have been shown to slow tumor growth for certain types of cancer. Who knew a crave-worthy burger could be so healthy?

INGREDIENTS

4 ounces ground turkey
¼ teaspoon garlic powder
⅛ teaspoon kosher salt
⅛ teaspoon black pepper
✪ 2 large portobello mushrooms, stems removed
1 tablespoon balsamic vinegar
1 tablespoon chopped red onion
1 basil leaf, thinly sliced
✪ 1 plum tomato, coarsely chopped
½ ounce sliced mozzarella

1. Combine turkey, garlic powder, salt, and pepper. Form into a patty.

2. Lightly oil and heat a grill or grill pan to medium-high. Cook burger and portobello caps, flipping once, until burger is cooked through and mushrooms are tender, 8 minutes.

3. Combine vinegar, onion, basil, and tomato. Season to taste with salt and pepper.

4. Using mushroom caps as buns, place burger inside and top with cheese and bruschetta mixture.

PER SERVING: 267 calories, 12 g fat (3.5 g saturated fat), 30 g protein, 341 mg sodium, 13 g carbohydrates, 9 g sugars (0 g added sugars), 3 g fiber

WEEKNIGHT DINNER

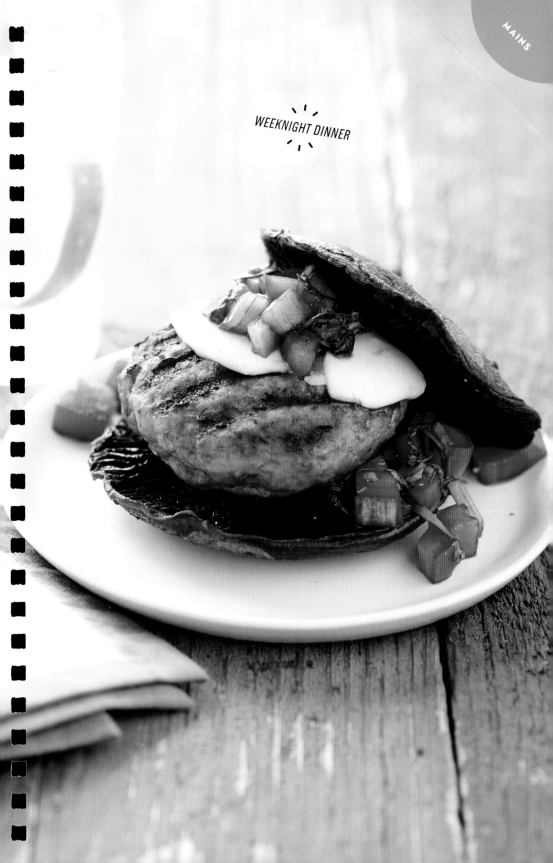

Thai Turkey Lettuce Cups with Cilantro Sauce

Active time: 20 minutes
Total time: 20 minutes
Makes: 4 servings

→ Cilantro has anti-inflammatory properties that help with arthritis. Lean ground turkey is a smart choice compared to lean ground beef, with about half the saturated fat. And lettuce cups are a great keto-friendly switch for bread, tortillas, or other carb-loaded options.

INGREDIENTS

CILANTRO SAUCE
1 jalapeño, seeded if desired, and chopped
✪ 2 tablespoons fresh lime juice
✪ ½ cup plain yogurt
1 cup cilantro leaves
½ teaspoon ground cumin

THAI TURKEY LETTUCE CUPS
1 tablespoon canola oil
1½ pounds lean white ground turkey
✪ 2 cloves garlic, finely chopped
1 jalapeño, finely chopped
1 tablespoon grated peeled fresh ginger
1 tablespoon coconut aminos
✪ 2 tablespoons lime juice
¼ cup water (optional)
2 scallions, thinly sliced
8 butter lettuce leaves
Sliced radishes, for serving (optional)

1. In a blender, puree jalapeño with lime juice, yogurt, cilantro, and cumin until very smooth. Set aside.

2. Heat canola oil in a large cast-iron skillet on medium-high. Add ground turkey and cook, breaking it up with a spoon, until golden brown and crispy, 6 to 8 minutes. Add garlic, jalapeño, and ginger and cook, tossing, for 1 minute.

3. Remove from heat and stir in coconut aminos, lime juice, and up to ¼ cup water if turkey mixture seems dry.

4. Sprinkle with scallions. Spoon into lettuce leaves and serve with cilantro sauce and sliced radishes, if desired.

PER SERVING: 250 calories, 6 g fat (1.5 g saturated fat), 43 g protein, 285 mg sodium, 5 g carbohydrates, 3 g sugars (0 g added sugars), 1 g fiber

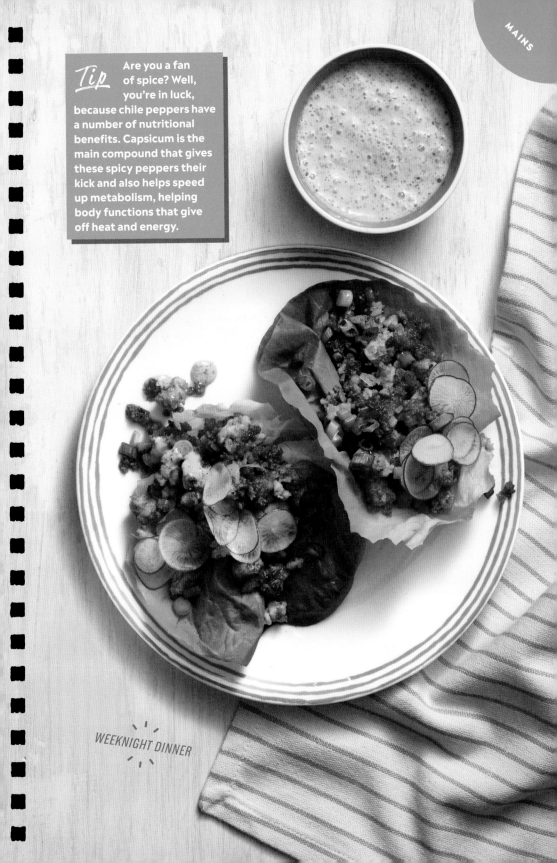

Tip Are you a fan of spice? Well, you're in luck, because chile peppers have a number of nutritional benefits. Capsicum is the main compound that gives these spicy peppers their kick and also helps speed up metabolism, helping body functions that give off heat and energy.

WEEKNIGHT DINNER

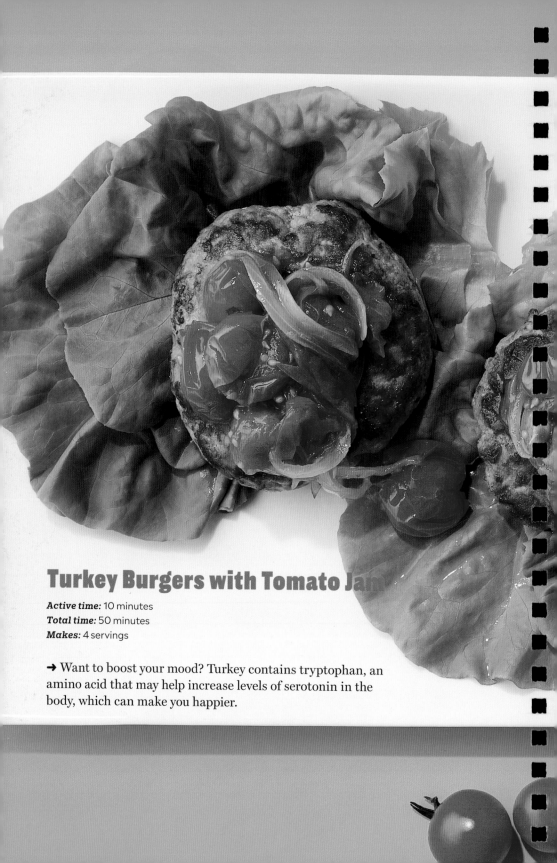

Turkey Burgers with Tomato Jam

Active time: 10 minutes
Total time: 50 minutes
Makes: 4 servings

→ Want to boost your mood? Turkey contains tryptophan, an amino acid that may help increase levels of serotonin in the body, which can make you happier.

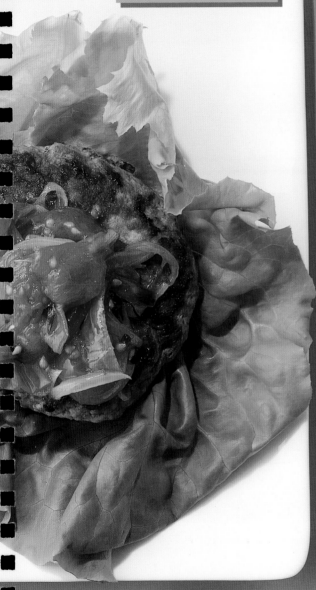

Tip Cooking tomatoes and onions brings out their natural sweetness and lets you skip ketchup, a sneaky source of added sugar.

INGREDIENTS

- ✪ 2 pints cherry tomatoes, halved
- ✪ 2 tablespoons olive oil
  1 teaspoon thyme leaves
- ✪ 4 cloves garlic
- ✪ 1 large sweet onion, thinly sliced
  ½ teaspoon salt
  ½ teaspoon black pepper
  1 pound ground turkey
- ✪ 4 leaves Bibb lettuce

1. Heat oven to 400°F. Toss tomatoes, 1 tablespoon olive oil, thyme, garlic, onion, and ¼ teaspoon each salt and pepper on a large rimmed baking sheet. Roast, stirring occasionally, until tomatoes are broken down, 35 minutes.

2. Meanwhile, season turkey with ¼ teaspoon each salt and pepper. Form 4 turkey patties. Heat 1 tablespoon olive oil in a large skillet on medium and cook burgers, flipping once, until cooked through, 10 minutes. Top each lettuce leaf with a burger.

3. Remove vegetables from oven. With a fork, mash garlic cloves. Toss vegetables to coat, lightly mashing mixture. Spoon 2 tablespoons tomato jam over each burger to serve.

PER SERVING: 223 calories, 13 g fat (3 g saturated fat), 23 g protein, 370 mg sodium, 4 g carbohydrates, 2 g sugars (0 g added sugars), 1 g fiber

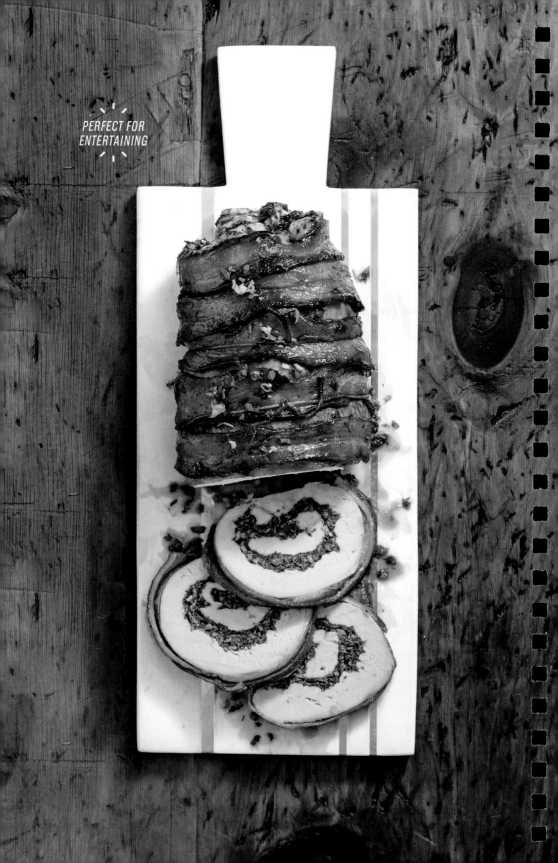

PERFECT FOR
ENTERTAINING

Glazed Bacon-Wrapped Turkey Breast

Active time: 20 minutes
Total time: 2 hours
Makes: 10 servings

→ Turkey breast is a healthy, low-fat, high-protein cut of meat that's full of vitamins. Wrapping the turkey breast in bacon helps to keep this delicious entrée keto friendly and the meat tender and moist.

INGREDIENTS

1 boneless turkey breast (4 to 5 pounds), skin removed
¾ teaspoon kosher salt
1½ bunches scallions, sliced
2 cups packed parsley leaves
✪ ⅓ cup olive oil
✪ 4 cloves garlic
12 ounces thick-cut bacon
4 cups water
¼ cup balsamic vinegar

1. Heat oven to 375°F. Line a roasting pan with foil.

2. Place turkey breast, smooth side down, on a cutting board. On the left breast, cut along the right side of the tenderloin to separate it from breast without cutting off the tenderloin; fold the tenderloin back. Repeat on the right breast, cutting along the left side of the tenderloin and folding it back. Cover surface of turkey with 3 large sheets of plastic wrap. With the flat side of a meat mallet or a heavy rolling pin, pound turkey until it is about 1 inch thick all over. Discard the plastic wrap.

3. Sprinkle surface of turkey with salt. In a food processor, pulse scallions, parsley, olive oil, and garlic until finely chopped, stopping to stir it occasionally. Spread herb mixture in an even layer on turkey breast. Starting at a short side, roll up the breast tightly. Place it seam side down on the cutting board. Drape bacon strips over turkey roll, overlapping the slices slightly. Tuck ends of bacon under turkey roll. Using 16-inch lengths of kitchen string, tie turkey tightly at 1½-inch intervals. (At this point, turkey may be wrapped tightly in plastic and refrigerated up to overnight.) Transfer turkey to a rack fitted into the prepared roasting pan. Add water to the bottom of the pan. Roast 45 minutes.

4. Brush vinegar over turkey, return pan to the oven, and roast another 45 minutes, or until turkey is cooked through (160°F), basting it with vinegar every 15 minutes. Remove turkey from the oven, loosely cover with foil, and let rest 20 minutes. Cut and discard the strings before slicing and serving.

PER SERVING:
About 380 calories, 15 g fat (4 g saturated fat), 54 g protein, 508 mg sodium, 4 g carbohydrates, 1 g sugars (0 g added sugars), 1 g fiber

Sausage & Pepper Bake

Active time: 10 minutes
Total time: 30 minutes
Makes: 4 servings

→ A take on a classic recipe uses turkey sausage to offer a healthy switch that is still full of protein but lower in calories, saturated fat, and sodium—can't say no to this one!

INGREDIENTS

2 bell peppers (orange, red, or a combination), halved and thickly sliced
- 1 pint cherry or grape tomatoes, halved
- 1 medium yellow onion, cut in 1-inch wedges
- 1 clove garlic, finely chopped
- 1 tablespoon olive oil
1 teaspoon dried oregano
Kosher salt and pepper
4 sweet or hot Italian turkey sausages (about 12 ounces), cut into 1½-inch pieces

1. Heat oven to 400°F. On a large rimmed baking sheet, toss bell peppers, tomatoes, onion, and garlic with olive oil, oregano, ¼ teaspoon salt, and ½ teaspoon pepper, then toss with sausages.

2. Roast until sausages are cooked through and beginning to blister and vegetables are golden brown and tender, 15 to 20 minutes.

PER SERVING: 210 calories, 13 g fat (0.5 g saturated fat), 16 g protein, 665 mg sodium, 10 g carbohydrates, 6 g sugars (0 g added sugars), 2 g fiber

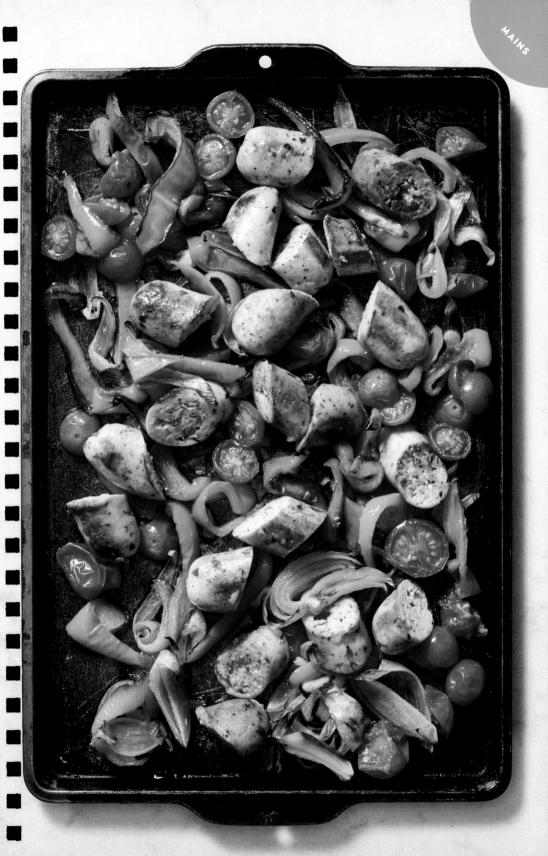

"Spaghetti" & Meatballs

Active time: 35 minutes
Total time: 40 minutes
Makes: 4 servings

→ Spiralized zucchini has become the new go-to as a carb substitute in so many recipes. Better yet, now most grocery stores sell zucchini already spiralized, reducing the prep work in this recipe!

INGREDIENTS

1 pound lean ground turkey
✪ ½ small onion, finely chopped
1 teaspoon dried oregano
1 teaspoon dried basil
1 teaspoon garlic powder
Kosher salt and pepper
✪ 1 tablespoon avocado oil or olive oil
✪ 1 24-ounce jar low-sodium marinara sauce
3 large zucchini (about 12 ounces each), spiralized into zoodles
¼ cup grated Parmesan, for serving

1. Heat broiler and line a rimmed baking sheet with nonstick foil.

2. In a large bowl, combine turkey, onion, oregano, basil, garlic powder, and ¼ teaspoon each salt and pepper. Roll into 28 balls, about 1 tablespoon each, and place on prepared baking sheet. Drizzle with oil and broil until cooked through, 6 to 8 minutes.

3. Meanwhile, in a large skillet, bring marinara sauce to a simmer. Add zoodles and simmer, tossing occasionally, until just tender, 5 to 7 minutes. Gently fold in meatballs and serve with Parmesan.

PER SERVING: 305 calories, 14 g fat (2 g saturated fat), 28 g protein, 450 mg sodium, 20 g carbohydates, 13 g sugars (3 g added sugars), 4 g fiber

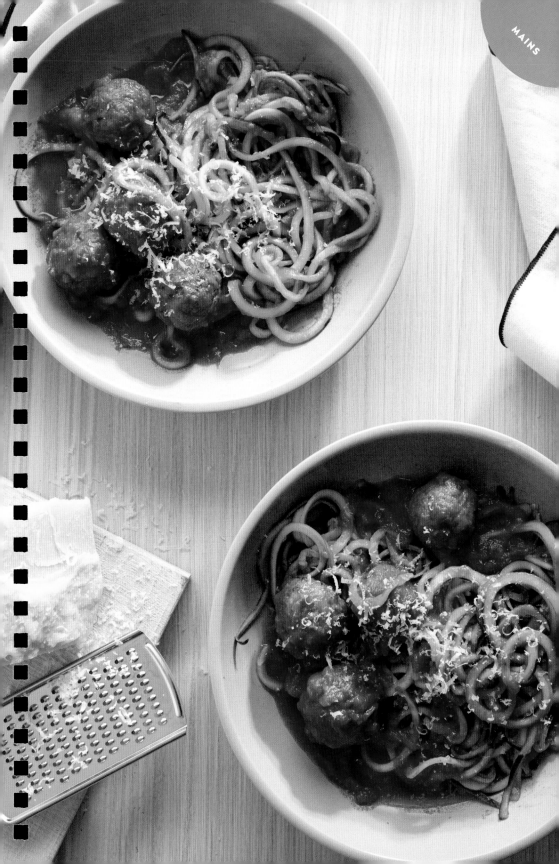

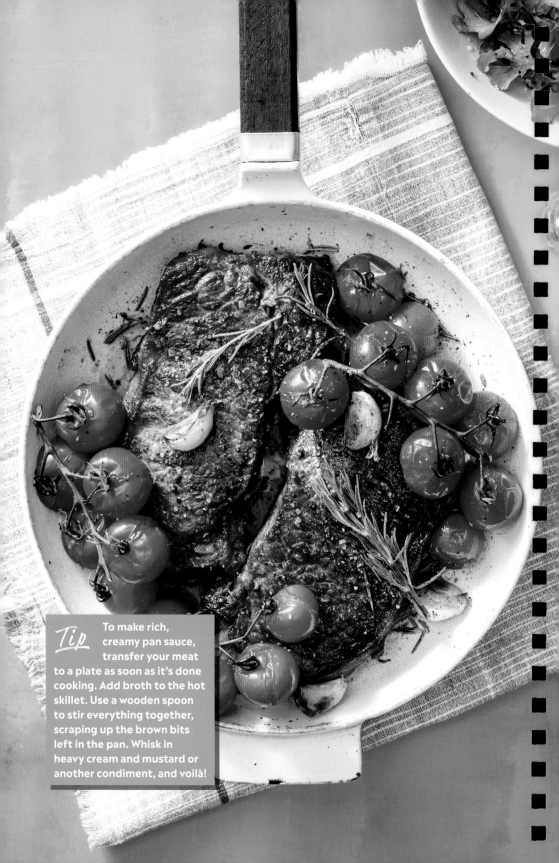

Tip To make rich, creamy pan sauce, transfer your meat to a plate as soon as it's done cooking. Add broth to the hot skillet. Use a wooden spoon to stir everything together, scraping up the brown bits left in the pan. Whisk in heavy cream and mustard or another condiment, and voilà!

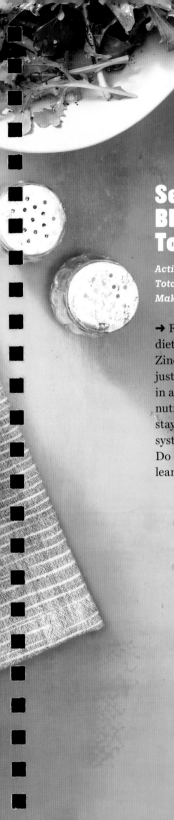

Seared Steak with Blistered Tomatoes

Active time: 5 minutes
Total time: 20 minutes
Makes: 4 servings

→ Red meat is important in the keto diet for its fat and vitamin content. Zinc, iron, and vitamin B12 are just some of the nutrients found in abundance in red meat. These nutrients help your red blood cells stay healthy and keep your immune system strong. The key is moderation: Do enjoy it, but when you can, choose lean beef varieties.

INGREDIENTS

2 strip steaks (about
 1½ pounds), each 1½
 inches thick
Kosher salt and ground
 black pepper
✪ 4 tablespoons olive oil
✪ 6 cloves garlic, unpeeled
✪ 2 bunches cherry tomatoes
 on the vine (about
 1½ pounds)
2 sprigs fresh rosemary
2 tablespoons white wine
 vinegar
✪ ¼ small red onion, finely
 chopped
3 tablespoons crumbled
 blue cheese (about
 1 ounce)
Arugula, for serving

1. Heat oven to 450°F. Heat a large oven-safe cast-iron skillet on medium-high. Season steaks with ¼ teaspoon each salt and pepper. Add 1 teaspoon olive oil to the skillet, then add steaks and garlic and cook until steaks are browned, 3 minutes per side.

2. Add tomatoes on the vine and rosemary to the skillet, drizzle with 2 teaspoons olive oil, and season with salt and pepper. Transfer skillet to the oven and roast until steak is at the desired degree of doneness, 3 to 4 minutes for medium-rare, and tomatoes begin to slightly break down. Transfer steaks to a cutting board and let rest at least 5 minutes before serving. Transfer tomatoes and garlic to a platter; squeeze garlic cloves from their skins.

3. In a small bowl, combine vinegar, 3 tablespoons olive oil, and ¼ teaspoon each salt and pepper; stir in onion and fold in blue cheese. Serve steak, tomatoes, and garlic alongside arugula drizzled with vinaigrette.

PER SERVING: About 445 calories, 28 g fat (8.5 g saturated fat), 39 g protein, 455 mg sodium, 9 g carbohydrates, 5 g sugars (0 g added sugars), 2g fiber

Feta and Mint Mini Meat Loaves with Squash

Active time: 15 minutes
Total time: 30 minutes
Makes: 4 servings

→ If you love the briny flavor of olives, these Greek meat loaves are perfect for your palate. Olives are part of the stone fruit family and are made up of 74 percent oleic acid, the healthy fatty acid that makes olive oil. This fatty acid helps to reduce inflammation, heart disease, and the risk of cancer—so many benefits in such a small bite!

INGREDIENTS
- ❌ 1¼ pounds ground beef chuck
- ½ cup crumbled feta cheese
- ½ cup mint leaves, finely chopped
- Kosher salt
- 1 large leek, sliced
- 3 medium yellow squash, chopped
- 1 cup pitted green olives
- ❌ 1 tablespoon olive oil

1. Heat oven to 450°F. In a bowl, combine beef chuck, feta, mint, and ¼ teaspoon salt. Divide mixture into fourths and form 4 mini loaves, placing them on a rimmed baking sheet.

2. In a separate bowl, toss leeks, squash, and olives with olive oil and ⅛ teaspoon salt; arrange vegetables around loaves on the baking sheet.

3. Roast until the meat loaves are cooked through (165°F), 15 to 20 minutes.

4. Serve meat loaves with vegetables.

PER SERVING: About 415 calories, 28 g fat (10 g saturated fat), 30 g protein, 935 mg sodium, 12 g carbohydrates, 5 g sugars (0 g added sugars), 4 g fiber

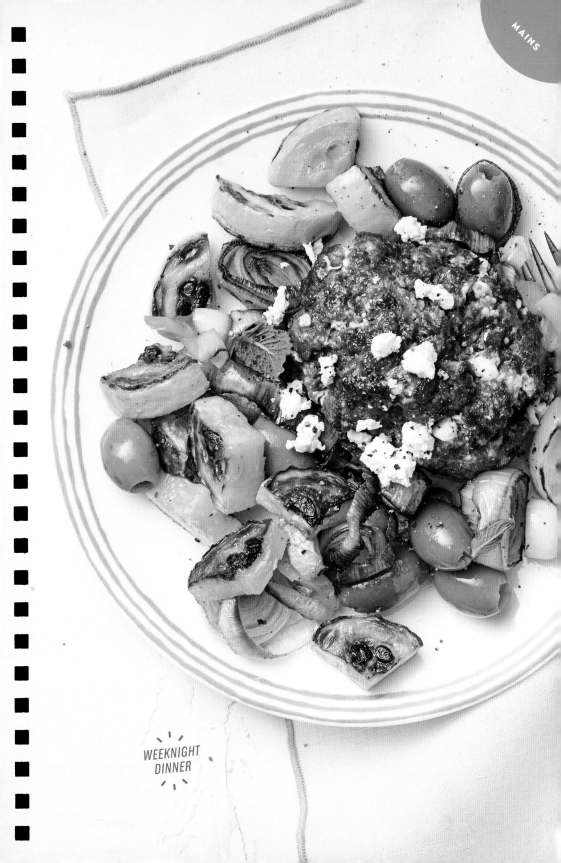

WEEKNIGHT
DINNER

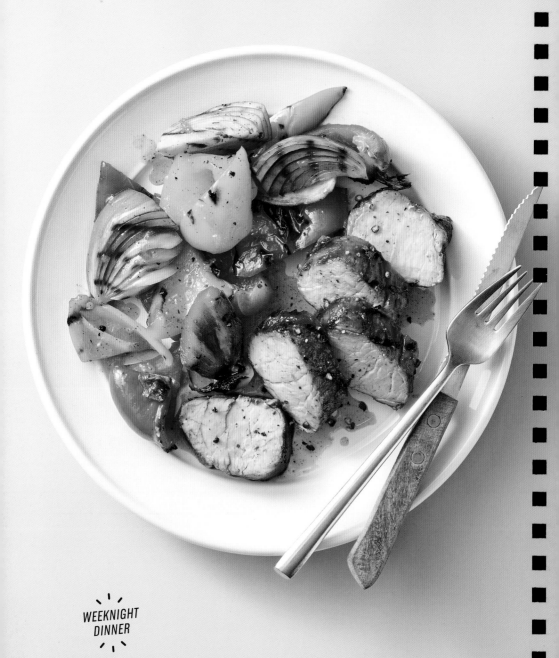

WEEKNIGHT
DINNER

Grilled Pork Tenderloin and Peppers

Active time: 10 minutes
Total time: 25 minutes
Makes: 4 servings

→ Sweet bell peppers are an excellent source of vitamin C. One pepper provides you 250 percent of your recommended daily value.

INGREDIENTS

- 4 bell peppers (red, yellow, orange, or a combination), quartered
- ✪ 1 red onion, cut into ½-inch wedges
- 1 tablespoon olive oil
- Kosher salt and ground black pepper
- 2 small pork tenderloins (about ¾ pound each)
- 2 tablespoons balsamic vinegar

1. Heat a grill on medium-high. In a bowl, toss bell peppers and red onion with olive oil and season to taste with salt and black pepper.

2. Season pork tenderloins with ¼ teaspoon each salt and black pepper. Cover and grill vegetables and pork, turning occasionally, until vegetables are tender, 8 to 10 minutes. Transfer vegetables to a cutting board.

3. Continue grilling pork, basting it with vinegar, until cooked through (145°F), 3 to 6 minutes. Let rest 5 minutes before slicing. Coarsely chop bell peppers and serve with onion and pork.

PER SERVING: About 275 calories, 9 g fat (2 g saturated fat), 36 g protein, 231 mg sodium, 12 g carbohydrates, 5 g sugars (0 g added sugars), 3 g fiber

Sausage-Stuffed Zucchini Boats

Active time: 20 minutes
Total time: 55 minutes
Makes: 4 servings

→ Marinara sauce is an easy store-bought solution, but many of these jarred sauces contain added sugars and other additives. Be sure to check the label for sneak ingredients or find a no-sugar-added or low-sugar marinara sauce to keep your carb count down.

INGREDIENTS
- 4 small zucchini
- ✪ 2 teaspoons olive oil
- ✪ 1 small onion, chopped
- 2 links sweet Italian sausage, casing removed
- ¼ teaspoon kosher salt
- ✪ 1¼ cups no-sugar-added marinara sauce
- 1 cup coarsely grated mozzarella
- Chopped parsley, for topping

1. Heat oven to 450°F.

2. Cut each zucchini in half lengthwise; scoop out and chop the flesh, leaving a ¼-inch shell.

3. Heat olive oil in a 10-inch skillet on medium-high. Add chopped zucchini, onion, Italian sausage, and salt. Cook 8 minutes, breaking up sausage with the back of a spoon.

4. In a 3-quart baking dish, spread marinara sauce evenly on the bottom; arrange zucchini shells on top, cut sides up. Spoon sausage mixture evenly into shells. Top with mozzarella. Cover dish with foil and bake 30 minutes. Uncover and bake 5 more minutes. Top with chopped parsley.

PER SERVING: About 325 calories, 23 g fat (9 g saturated fat), 16 g protein, 925 mg sodium, 15 g carbohydrates, 7 g sugars (0 g added sugars), 3 g fiber

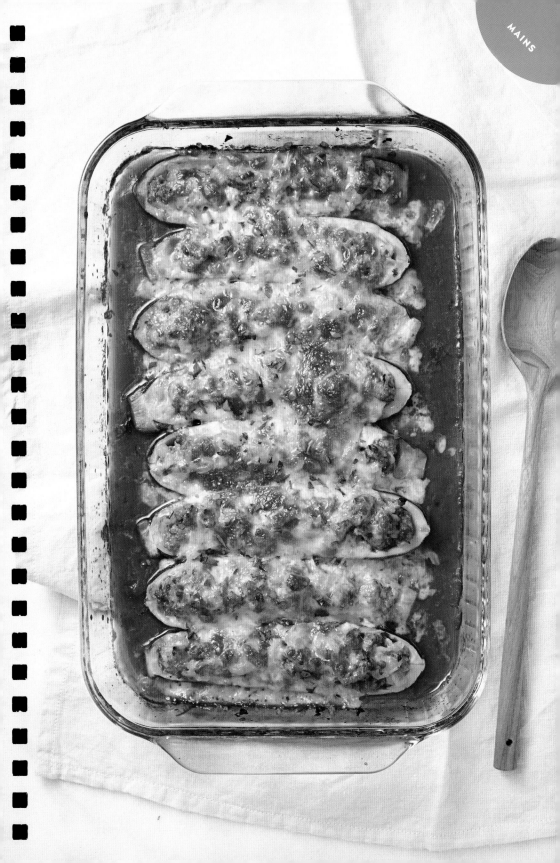

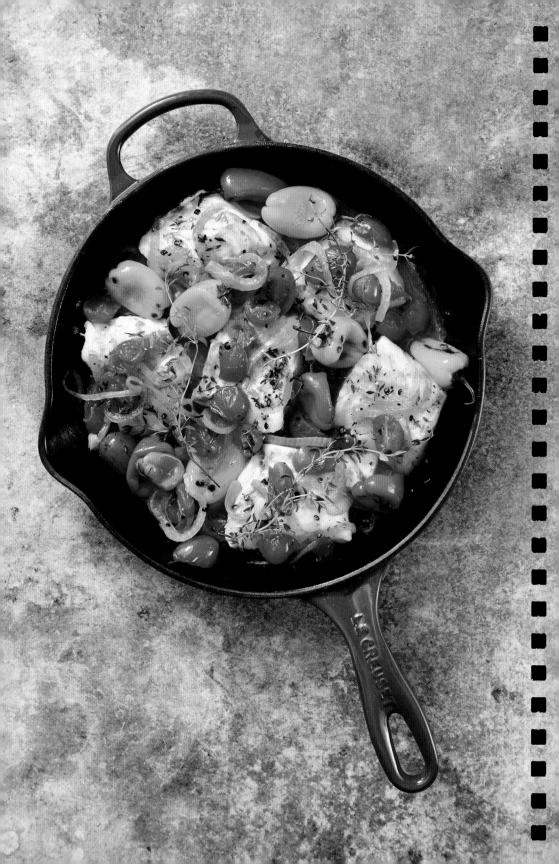

Mediterranean Baked Cod

Active time: 10 minutes
Total time: 25 minutes
Makes: 4 servings

→ Selenium and phosphorous are two important minerals found in cod. Selenium helps form and protect your DNA, while phosphorous is critical for good teeth and bone health.

INGREDIENTS

- ✪ 1 tablespoon olive oil
- ✪ 1 medium onion, thinly sliced
- 6 ounces mini sweet peppers, halved lengthwise
- Kosher salt
- ✪ 1 pint grape tomatoes, halved lengthwise
- 8 sprigs fresh thyme
- ✪ 1½ pounds cod fillets
- ¼ cup water
- ¼ teaspoon ground black pepper

1. Heat oven to 450°F.

2. Heat olive oil in a 7- to 8-quart wide-bottomed oven-safe pot on medium-high. Add onion, sweet peppers, and ¼ teaspoon salt and cook, stirring occasionally, until onions are almost tender, 5 minutes.

3. Add grape tomatoes and thyme; cook 2 minutes.

4. Add cod fillets and water; sprinkle cod with ¼ teaspoon each salt and the pepper. Cover and bake until cod is cooked through, 15 minutes. Discard thyme sprigs and serve.

PER SERVING:
About 205 calories, 5 g fat (1 g saturated fat), 32 g protein, 115 mg sodium, 8 g carbohydrates, 4 g sugars (0 g added sugars), 1 g fiber

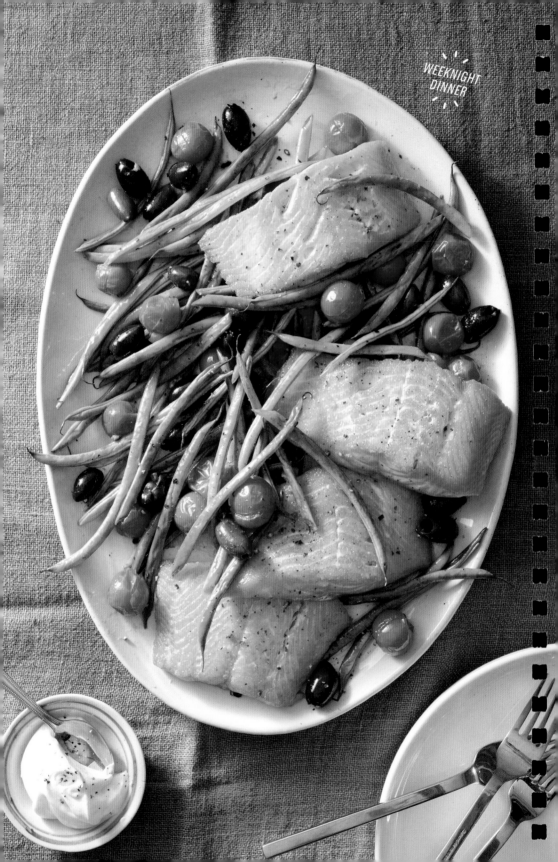

Roasted Salmon with Tomatoes and Green Beans

Active time: 5 minutes
Total time: 25 minutes
Makes: 2 servings

→ Salmon is a keto superhero. Rich in healthy fats like omega-3s, and a good source of protein, it's also satisfying and versatile.

INGREDIENTS

6 ounces green beans, trimmed
¼ cup water
✪ 1 cup grape tomatoes
¼ cup pitted kalamata olives
✪ 4 oil-packed anchovies, drained
✪ 1 tablespoon olive oil
Kosher salt and ground black pepper
✪ 2 6-ounce skinless center-cut salmon fillets

1. Heat oven to 425°F. Heat a large oven-safe skillet on medium-high, add green beans and water, cover, and cook, shaking the pan occasionally, 3 minutes. Drain beans and transfer to a bowl.

2. Wipe out the skillet. Toss beans in bowl with grape tomatoes, olives, anchovies, and olive oil and lightly season with salt and pepper. Transfer mixture to the skillet and roast 8 minutes.

3. Season salmon fillets with salt and pepper and nestle them among vegetables in the skillet. Roast until salmon is just opaque throughout, 10 to 12 minutes.

PER SERVING: About 355 calories, 18 g fat (3.5 g saturated fat), 38 g protein, 1,105 mg sodium, 10 g carbohydrates, 4 g sugars (0 g added sugars), 4 g fiber

Garlicky Mussels with Green Bean "Fries"

Active time: 10 minutes
Total time: 20 minutes
Makes: 4 servings

→ If you are a fan of mussels, then you are in luck. Not only are they big in flavor, but they also contain vitamin B12, a key nutrient that supports nerve and red blood cell health.

INGREDIENTS

- 12 ounces green beans, trimmed
- ✪ 2 tablespoons olive oil
- Salt and pepper
- ✪ 3 large cloves garlic, finely chopped
- ¾ cup dry white wine
- ✪ 4 pounds mussels, scrubbed
- ✪ 2 beefsteak tomatoes, chopped
- ¼ cup flat-leaf parsley, chopped

1. On a rimmed baking sheet, toss green beans with 1 tablespoon olive oil and ¼ teaspoon each salt and pepper; broil until just tender, about 7 minutes.

2. Heat a large Dutch oven on medium. Add 1 tablespoon olive oil, garlic, and a pinch of salt, then sauté 30 seconds.

3. Add white wine and bring to a boil. Add mussels and simmer, covered, stirring twice, until shells open, 5 to 8 minutes. Discard any unopened shells.

4. Toss cooked mussels with tomatoes and parsley. Serve with green beans.

PER SERVING: 220 calories, 10 g fat (1.5 g saturated fat), 16 g protein, 485 mg sodium, 17 g carbohydrates, 6 g sugars (0 g added sugars), 4 g fiber

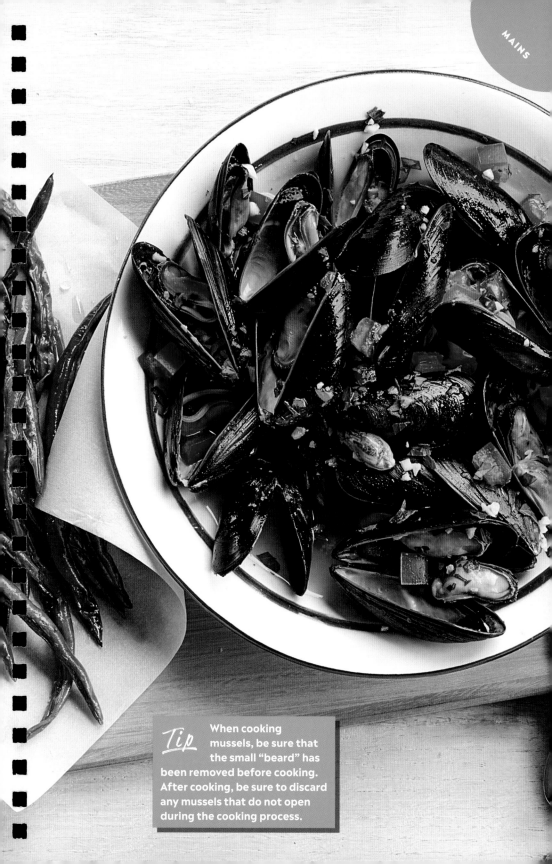

Tip When cooking mussels, be sure that the small "beard" has been removed before cooking. After cooking, be sure to discard any mussels that do not open during the cooking process.

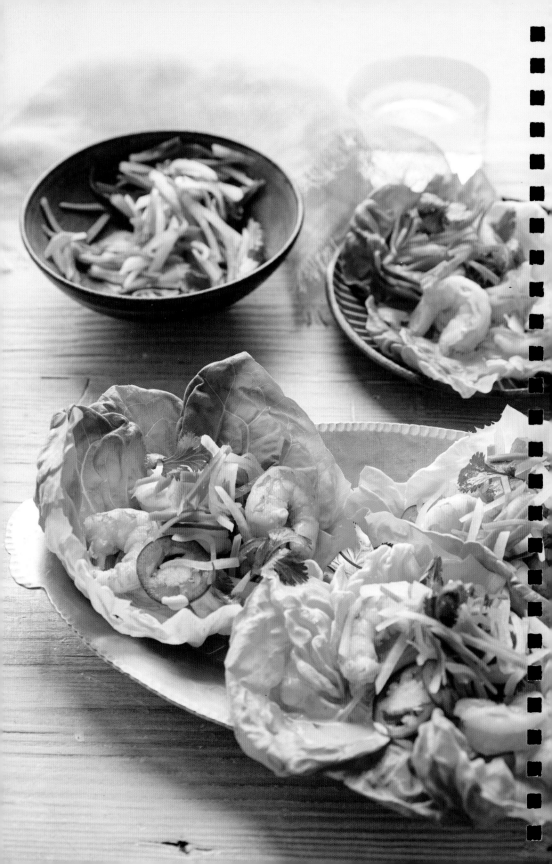

Spicy Shrimp Tacos

Active time: 10 minutes
Total time: 25 minutes
Makes: 4 servings

→ Flavored with a zesty mayo-based spread and cool pickled vegetables, these shrimp tacos have twice the protein that's in a fried-fish taco. Wrapped in a lettuce leaf, they are low-carb, too!

INGREDIENTS
⅓ cup white wine vinegar
1 teaspoon grated ginger
½ teaspoon kosher salt
½ cup grated carrot
½ cup grated daikon radish
¼ cup mayonnaise
2 teaspoons sriracha
1 teaspoon coconut aminos
✪ 4 large leaves of butter lettuce
✪ 12 ounces medium shrimp, cooked, peeled, and deveined
1 jalapeño, thinly sliced
2 tablespoons cilantro leaves, for topping

1. Stir together ⅓ cup hot water, vinegar, ginger, and salt in a medium bowl. Submerge carrot and radish; let sit 10 minutes.

2. Mix mayonnaise, sriracha, and coconut aminos in a small bowl. Spread over lettuce leaves. Add shrimp and jalapeño. Top with pickled carrot-radish mixture and sprinkle with cilantro.

PER SERVING: 163 calories, 10 g fat (1.5 g saturated fat), 13 g protein, 475 mg sodium, 4 g carbohydrates, 2 g sugars (0 g added sugars), 1 g fiber

Parchment-Baked Halibut with Fennel and Carrots

Active time: 10 minutes
Total time: 35 minutes
Makes: 4 servings

→ Cooking foods in parchment paper, or *en papillote*, creates a small packet where the food is allowed to steam in its own juices. Fish cooks perfectly with this easy steam method. In this case, halibut is an ideal flaky fish option, plus it contains selenium, an antioxidant that helps with inflammation and repairing cells.

INGREDIENTS

1 bulb fennel, cored, thinly sliced, fronds reserved
½ bunch young carrots, quartered, tops removed
1 small shallot, sliced
✪ 4 6-ounce skinless halibut fillets
½ teaspoon kosher salt
¼ teaspoon black pepper
✪ 4 slices orange
8 sprigs thyme
4 leaves fresh sage, sliced
½ cup white wine

1. Heat oven to 425°F. Tear 4 squares of parchment paper, each about 15 by 15 inches.

2. In the center of a piece of parchment, set ¼ of fennel, carrots, and shallot, topped by 1 piece of fish. Sprinkle with ⅛ teaspoon salt and a pinch of pepper. Lay 1 slice orange, 2 sprigs thyme, ¼ sage leaves, and a bit of fennel frond on top. Drizzle 2 tablespoons wine around fish.

3. Bring up opposite sides of the parchment and fold them together, as if you were folding the top of a paper bag, to seal all edges. Set packet on a rimmed baking sheet and repeat with remaining ingredients.

4. Bake until packets are slightly browned and puffed, about 13 minutes. Let rest 2 to 3 minutes. Set individual packets on plates, and with kitchen shears or a small knife, carefully cut open at the table. (Caution: Escaping steam will be hot.)

PER SERVING: 253 calories, 3 g fat (0.5 g saturated fat), 34 g protein, 455 mg sodium, 18 g carbohydrates, 7 g sugars (0 g added sugars), 5 g fiber

Tip Did you know that just a half-fillet of halibut has more than a third of your daily needs for several vitamins and minerals? Selenium, phosphorous, and vitamins B12 and B6 are just a couple of examples. This fish is also a perfect mild base to pair with any spice or herb, making it a winner for both taste and nutrition!

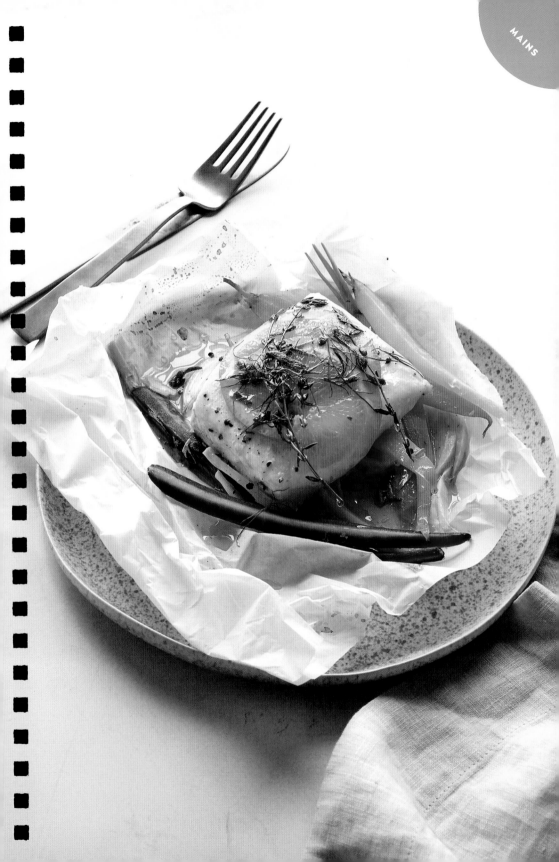

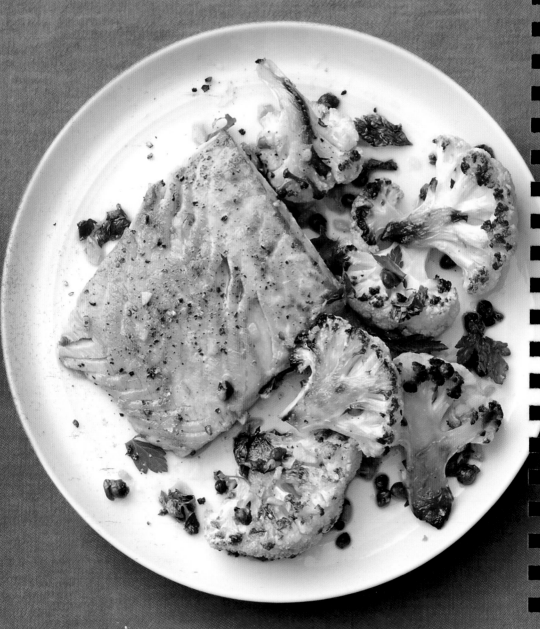

WEEKNIGHT
DINNER

Seared Salmon with Roasted Cauliflower

Active time: 10 minutes
Total time: 30 minutes
Makes: 4 servings

→ They may be small, but briny capers bring a strong finishing flavor and a surprisingly healthy punch to many recipes. They are a heart-healthy ingredient that may even help fight cancer, thanks to their rich antioxidants.

INGREDIENTS
1½ pounds cauliflower florets (1 large head of cauliflower)
★ Olive oil
Salt and pepper
★ 4 6-ounce salmon fillets
★ 2 cloves garlic, chopped
1 tablespoon capers
½ cup parsley leaves, chopped

1. Heat oven to 450°F. On a rimmed baking sheet, toss cauliflower florets with 2 tablespoons olive oil and ¼ teaspoon each salt and pepper.

2. Roast cauliflower until tender, then broil until golden brown, about 3 minutes. Let cool.

3. Season salmon to taste with salt and pepper. Heat 2 teaspoons olive oil in a large skillet on medium-high. Cook salmon until opaque throughout, 8 to 9 minutes, adding garlic and capers to the skillet after flipping the salmon once. Remove salmon from heat and set aside while preparing cauliflower.

4. Toss cauliflower with capers, garlic, and parsley. Serve with salmon.

PER SERVING: 305 calories, 15.5 g fat (3 g saturated fat), 36 g protein, 400 mg sodium, 5 g carbohydrates, 1 g sugars (0 g added sugars), 2 g fiber

Chapter 5

Sides

Side dishes help to round out any meal that seems a little light. Plus, the selections in this chapter are packed with healthy vegetables to add extra vitamins and minerals to your daily keto diet. Eating these vegetables at their peak harvest time will assure the most vibrant natural flavor. Try the Sautéed Spinach with Garlic (or substitute any dark leafy green) in the summer or Brussels Sprouts with Bacon in the winter. Asparagus with Egg Mimosa is a delight in the spring. Once you understand the general technique of each recipe, you'll see that each of these side dishes can be made with different vegetables depending on what's in season, your mood, or the other dishes on the table. So now there really isn't any excuse not to eat your veggies!

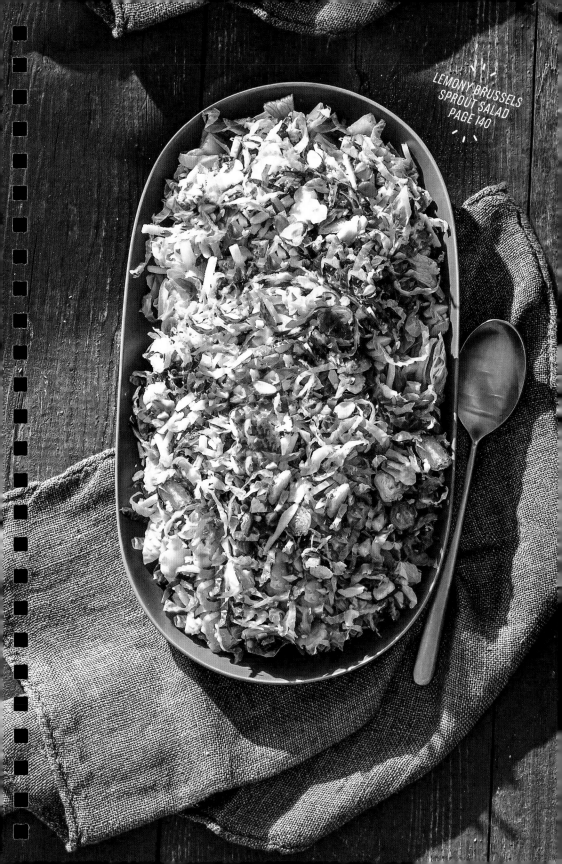

LEMONY BRUSSELS
SPROUT SALAD
PAGE 140

Turkish Shepherd's Salad

Active time: 15 minutes
Total time: 15 minutes
Makes: 6 servings

➜ Herbs can take even the freshest salad to the next level in flavor. The triple-threat combination of parsley, mint, and dill brightens the garden flavors as well as the health benefits of this dish. Parsley can help stimulate appetite and soothe irritated skin. Some of dill's healing properties include treatment for fever, colds, cough, infections, menstrual cramps, and sleep disorders. Mint's benefits range from improving brain function to relieving breastfeeding pain, cold symptoms, and even bad breath. Plus, all three herbs aid in digestion, which is important when eating lots of high-fat foods.

INGREDIENTS

- ★ ¼ cup extra-virgin olive oil
- 2 tablespoons cider vinegar
- ★ 2 tablespoons lemon juice
- ½ teaspoon kosher salt
- ¼ teaspoon black pepper
- ★ 3 plum tomatoes, seeded and chopped
- 2 cucumbers, seeded and chopped
- 1 red bell pepper, chopped
- 1 green bell pepper, chopped
- ★ 1 small red onion, chopped
- ⅓ cup pitted black olives (such as kalamata), halved
- ½ cup chopped flat-leaf parsley
- ¼ cup chopped mint leaves
- ¼ cup chopped dill leaves
- 6 ounces feta cheese, cubed, for topping

1. In a small bowl, whisk together olive oil, vinegar, lemon juice, salt, and black pepper.

2. In a large serving bowl, combine tomatoes, cucumbers, bell peppers, onions, olives, parsley, mint, and dill. Pour dressing over salad, toss gently, and top with cheese.

PER SERVING: 238 calories, 20 g fat (6 g saturated fat), 6 g protein, 806 mg sodium, 10 g carbohydrates, 5 g sugars (0 g added sugars), 2 g fiber

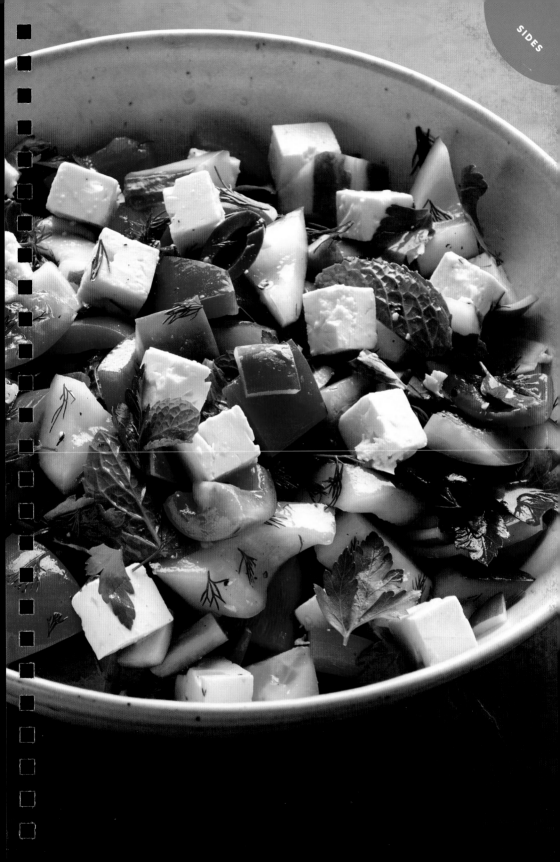

Lemony Brussels Sprout Salad

Active time: 20 minutes
Total time: 25 minutes
Makes: 8 servings

→ Brussels sprouts are tiny but mighty nutritional powerhouses. Like their cruciferous cousins (broccoli, cabbage, and cauliflower) they deliver more than 100 percent of the recommended daily allowance for vitamins C and K, a healthy dose of fiber, and antioxidants.

INGREDIENTS

- ✪ ¼ cup fresh lemon juice
- ✪ 3 tablespoons extra-virgin olive oil
- ½ teaspoon kosher salt
- ¼ teaspoon ground black pepper
- ✪ 1 pound Brussels sprouts, trimmed and very thinly sliced
- ✪ 1 small head romaine lettuce, chopped
- ⅓ cup packed grated ricotta salata or Pecorino Romano cheese
- ✪ ½ cup smoked almonds, chopped

1. In a large bowl, whisk together lemon juice, oil, salt, and pepper; add Brussels sprouts and toss until well coated. Let stand at least 10 minutes or up to 2 hours.

2. When ready to serve, add romaine, ricotta salata, and almonds to the bowl with Brussels sprouts; toss to combine.

PER SERVING: 145 calories, 12 g fat (2 g saturated fat), 5 g protein, 292 mg sodium, 8 g carbohydrates, 1 g sugars (0 g added sugar), 3 g fiber

Tip The easiest way to thinly shave Brussels sprouts is on a mandolin. Leave the stem on and, holding the stem, carefully slice from top toward the stem. You can also use the food processor; simply pile trimmed sprouts into the feed tube.

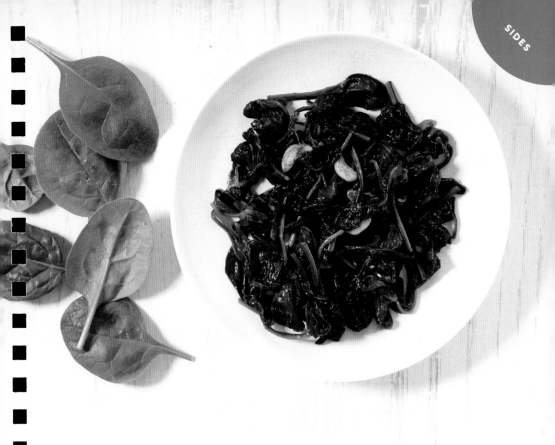

Sautéed Spinach with Garlic

Active time: 5 minutes
Total time: 10 minutes
Makes: 4 servings

→ Here's an easy side dish that you can make with any leafy green to meet your quotas of vitamins A, K, and C as well as calcium, magnesium, and potassium. If you like a bit of heat, add ¼ teaspoon red pepper flakes along with the garlic.

INGREDIENTS

- ✪ 1 tablespoon olive oil
- ✪ 2 cloves garlic, crushed with the side of a chef's knife
- ✪ 2 10-ounce bags fresh spinach, well rinsed
- ✪ 1 tablespoon fresh lemon juice
- ¼ teaspoon kosher salt

1. Heat olive oil in a 5- to 6-quart pot on medium-high until hot. Add garlic and cook, stirring continuously, until golden, about 1 minute.

2. Add spinach, with water clinging to the leaves, to the pot in 2 or 3 batches; cook until all the spinach fits in the pot, about 2 minutes. Cover and cook, stirring once, just until spinach wilts, 2 to 3 minutes. Remove from the heat. Stir in lemon juice and salt.

PER SERVING: About 45 calories, 4 g fat (1 g saturated fat), 4 g protein, 305 mg sodium, 1 g carbohydrates, 1 g sugars (0 g added sugars), 12 g fiber

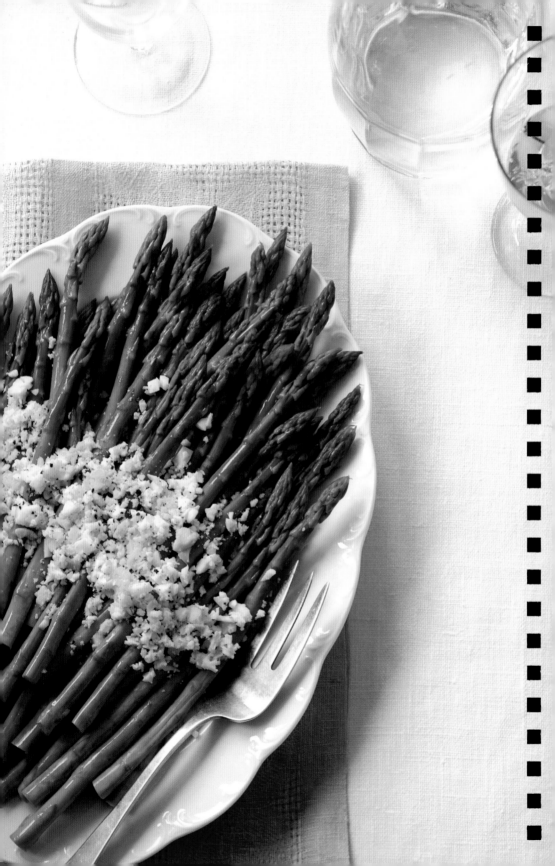

Asparagus with Egg Mimosa

Active time: 20 minutes
Total time: 35 minutes
Makes: 6 servings

→ This springtime vegetable is a member of the lily family and contains iron, zinc, and vitamin K. It's also a great source of folate, which is essential to cell growth and formation of DNA

INGREDIENTS
- ✪ 3 large eggs
- 2 pounds asparagus, trimmed
- ¼ cup water
- ✪ 1 lemon
- ✪ 3 tablespoons extra-virgin olive oil
- 2 tablespoons red wine vinegar
- 1 tablespoon snipped fresh chives
- ½ teaspoon kosher salt
- ½ teaspoon ground black pepper

1. In a 2-quart saucepan, combine eggs and enough cold water to cover. Bring water to a boil on high. Remove pan from heat, cover, and let stand 14 minutes. Rinse eggs under cold water until cool, then peel. Eggs may be hard-boiled and refrigerated up to 3 days ahead.

2. Meanwhile, arrange asparagus in an even layer in a microwave-safe 8-inch square baking dish. Add water. Cover with vented plastic wrap and microwave on High 5 minutes. Asparagus may be cooked, cooled, and refrigerated in an airtight container up to 2 days ahead.

3. From the lemon, grate ¼ teaspoon zest; set aside. Squeeze 1 tablespoon juice into a small bowl. Add olive oil, vinegar, chives, salt, and pepper; whisk to combine.

4. To serve, arrange asparagus on a serving platter. Drizzle with vinaigrette. Coarsely grate hard-boiled eggs over asparagus and top with reserved lemon zest.

PER SERVING: About 135 calories, 11 g total fat (2 g saturated fat), 6 g protein, 255 mg sodium, 3 g carbohydrates, 1 g sugars (0 g added sugars), 2 g fiber

Brussels Sprouts with Bacon

Active time: 15 minutes
Total time: 40 minutes
Makes: 10 servings

→ Brussels sprouts are part of the family of cruciferous vegetables that contain a cancer-reducing sulfur compound called glucosinolates. They are also high in iron, potassium, and folate, which are good for digestion and healthy red blood cells.

INGREDIENTS

2 quarts water
✪ 3 10-ounce containers Brussels sprouts, trimmed and cut in half lengthwise
6 slices bacon
1 tablespoon olive oil
✪ 2 cloves garlic, finely chopped
½ teaspoon salt
¼ teaspoon coarsely ground black pepper
✪ ¼ cup pine nuts, toasted, for topping

1. In a 4-quart saucepan, bring water to a boil on high. Add Brussels sprouts, return water to a boil, and cook until Brussels sprouts are tender-crisp, about 5 minutes; drain.

2. In a 12-inch skillet, cook bacon on medium until browned. With tongs, transfer bacon to paper towels to drain and cool; crumble.

3. Discard all but 1 tablespoon bacon drippings from the skillet. Add olive oil and heat on medium-high. Add Brussels sprouts, garlic, salt, and pepper. Cook, stirring frequently, until Brussels sprouts are lightly browned, about 5 minutes. Top with pine nuts and bacon.

PER SERVING: About 95 calories, 6 g fat (1 g saturated fat), 5 g protein, 200 mg sodium, 8 g carbohydrates, 2 g sugars (0 g added sugars), 3 g fiber

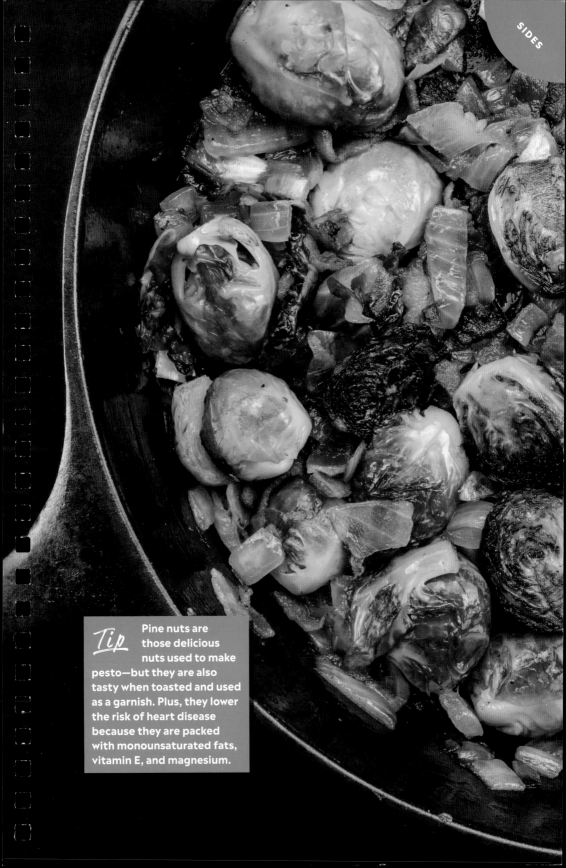

Tip Pine nuts are those delicious nuts used to make pesto—but they are also tasty when toasted and used as a garnish. Plus, they lower the risk of heart disease because they are packed with monounsaturated fats, vitamin E, and magnesium.

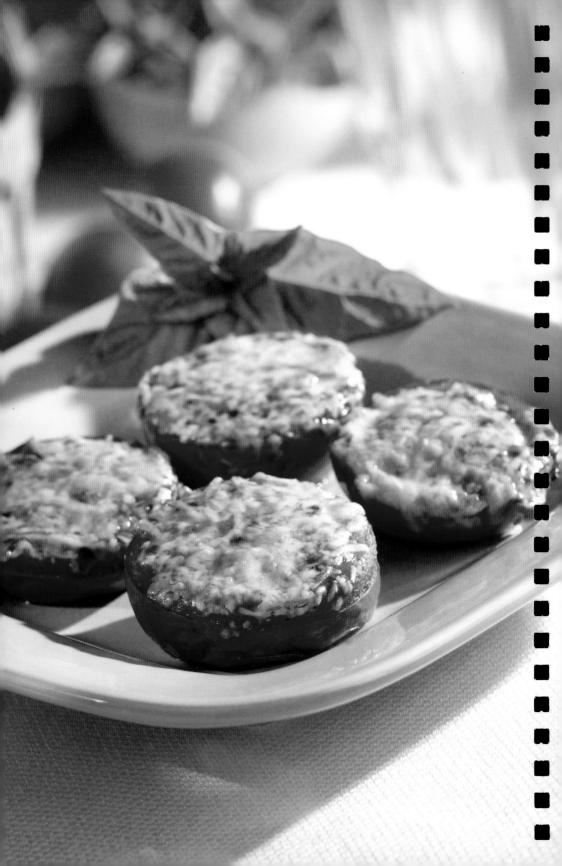

Broiled Parmesan Tomatoes

Active time: 10 minutes
Total time: 15 minutes
Makes: 4 servings

→ If you're not usually a fan of raw tomatoes, try them broiled. A direct blast of heat brings out the natural sweetness of the fruit along with a little bit of charred flavor. Topping the tomatoes with cheese makes them even more delicious!

INGREDIENTS

1 tablespoon butter
✪ 1 clove garlic, finely chopped
¼ cup freshly grated Parmesan
✪ 4 small ripe plum tomatoes (3 ounces each), cut in half lengthwise

1. Heat broiler. Melt butter in a 1-quart saucepan on low. Add garlic and cook, stirring, until golden; remove from heat.

2. Scatter Parmesan on a sheet of waxed paper. Dip the cut sides of tomatoes in garlic butter, then in Parmesan; place tomatoes, cheese side up, on a wire rack set in the broiler pan. Sprinkle any remaining Parmesan on top; drizzle with any remaining garlic butter.

3. Place the pan under the broiler at the closest position to the heat source. Broil until Parmesan is golden, 3 to 4 minutes.

PER SERVING: About 70 calories, 5 g fat (3 g saturated fat), 3 g protein, 150 mg sodium, 4 g carbohydrates, 2 g sugars (0 g added sugars), 1g fiber

147

INDEX

Note: Page numbers in *italics* indicate photos separate from recipes.

PHOTO CREDITS

COVER:
Danielle Daly.
Food Stylist: Cyd McDowell.
Prop Stylist: Alex Mata.

Sang An 54, 70
Beatriz DaCosta 126
Danielle Daly 23, 81, 116, 120
Phillip Ficks 35
Phillip Friedman 82, 98, 115
Mike Garten 37, 38, 42, 46, 52, 56, 65, 79, 102, 107, 110, 119, 123, 124,137

Getty Images 7 A. Namenko, 11 Nattakorn Maneerat, 13 Eugene Mymrin,
15 measuring cups: Elenathewise; food processor: Don Nichols; knife:
George Mdvanian/EyeEm; spiralizer: Olga Miltsova; blender: Pakorn
Kumruen/EyeEm, 16 Yagi Studio, 17 salmon: Aleimage; beef: Ahirao_
photo; chicken: JLDeines, 18-19 chia: Stockcam; avocado: Turnervisual;
kale: slyudmila; brussels sprouts: Creativeye 99; spinach: Slavko Sereda;
garlic: esseffe; onions: xxmmxx; tomato: mbbirdy, 20-21 orange: Philippe
Desnerck; almonds: Sirinate Kaewma/EyeEm; eggs: stockcam; yogurt:
phive2015; mushrooms: ansonsaw; olive oil: Anthony Rosenberg,
26 tashka2000, 29 Tetra Images, 33 Pinkybird, 45 Diana Miller, 61
fcafotodigital, 63 nevodka, 83 shaunl, 99 PlaniView, 103 chili peppers:
Manny R/Blend Images LLC; grapefruit: JamieB, 141 Slavko Sereda, 145
Kelly VanDellen, 146 Paul Poplis

Erika LaPresto 134
Bobbi Lin 66, 108
Mitch Mandel 85, 101, 105, 133, 139
Kate Mathis 86
Susan Pittard 27
Con Poulos 31, 41, 72, 76, 89, 129, 130
Armando Rafael 74
Travis Rathbone 44, 50
Kate Sears 142
Shutterstock 103 chives: Ines Behrens-Kunkel; tomato paste: Volosina
Christopher Testani 69, 90, 93, 97, 113
Jason Varney 28, 48

HEARST
HOME

Cover design by Made Visible Studio
Book design by Made Visible Studio

Library of Congress Cataloging-in-Publication Data Available on Request

10 9 8 7 6 5 4 3 2 1

Published by Hearst Home, an imprint of Hearst Books/Hearst Magazine Media, Inc.
Hearst Magazine Media, Inc.
300 West 57th Street
New York, NY 10019

Hearst Home, the Hearst Home logo, and Hearst Books are registered trademarks of Hearst Magazine Media, Inc.
Prevention is a registered trademark of Hearst Magazines, Inc

For information about custom editions, special sales, premium and corporate purchases, please go to hearst.com/magazines/hearst-books

Printed in China
ISBN 978-1-950785-05-6